# The Science, Art and Future of Spirit Healing

*Books by Paul Miller*

BORN TO HEAL
SCIENCE IN THE SEANCE ROOM
FACES OF THE LIVING DEAD
THE WAR DEAD RETURN
CAVALCADE OF THE SPIRIT
THE CHURCH IN DECAY
ORTHODOXY, THE ENEMY OF MANKIND

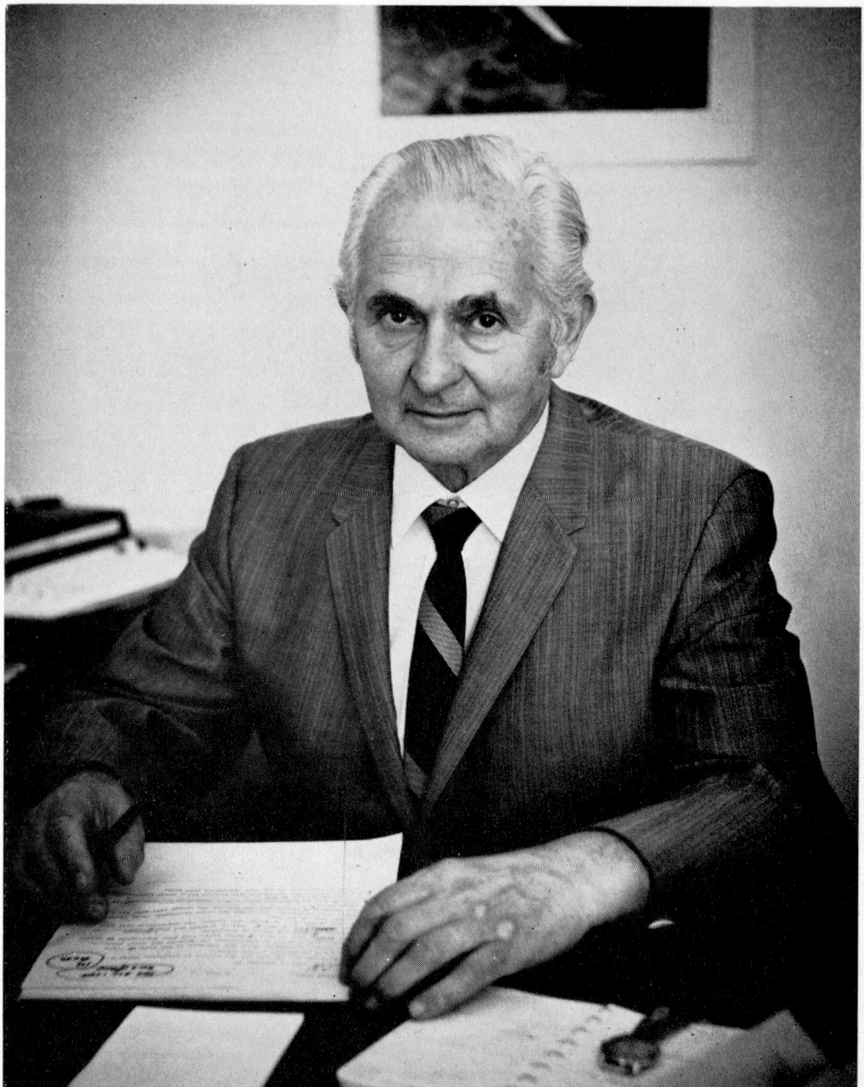

PAUL MILLER

# THE SCIENCE, ART and FUTURE of SPIRIT HEALING

by

PAUL MILLER

*in collaboration with Harry Edwards*

Published by
The Healer Publishing Company Limited
Burrows Lea, Shere, Guildford, Surrey

## AUTHOR'S NOTE

Many wonder about the source and nature of their inspiration and silent instruction.

If this book lightens their understanding, all is well.

To those who serve without thought of personal reward I offer this encouragement; there is light within the darkness and joy beyond telling when we bring knowledge of the spiritual life to others on the way.

And to my 'friend and counsellor', Harry Edwards, gratitude for healing so many who never saw him nor heard his voice.



Printed in Great Britain by The Anchor Press Ltd
and bound by Wm Brendon & Son Ltd
both of Tiptree, Essex

## CONTENTS

## LIST OF PLATES

# INTRODUCTION

Increasing Evidence for Survival of Bodily Death

Increasing Proof of Spirit Healing

All Humanity Comprised of Spirit Beings

Life is Continuous as Evolution is Continuous

Spirit Healing Mission Changing Human Thought

This is a prophetic work, not in the sense of foretelling specific events to occur at specific times and in specific conditions. It is intended to show that because we know something of the road travelled so far, it is reasonable to assume that we will continue in the same direction or will change direction until we have either achieved some awareness of a destiny or reach a roadblock of despair. What that destiny is, in principle, we cannot know now in precise form or condition but we are impelled towards it because we cannot go backwards in evolution.

There must be a destiny, not a destination, because life itself is eternal and from that we cannot retreat or flee. In the scientific field much that is to come is foreshadowed in what is already known. It is not the "same as before" prescription since nothing is the same absolutely from moment to moment. We advance from one frontier of knowledge to another. We turn to our memories daily to discuss with one another the differences between what is now and what was in our earlier years. In material changes alone, we wonder: what comes next?

In our wondering there is uncertainty: where will all this change—and much decay—lead us? There are many prophets, although called by other names, who tell us in many publications and orations what is to come. Some of it is frightening, if you are pessimistic by nature. Some is encouraging, if you are optimistic, but all of it speaks of change, change, change.

If so much is changing so much, what is permanent? Life alone is permanent. That is one certainty. Yet, within life there is unending variation until it seems to come to this basic consideration: we all come here, we have many experiences, we are sad and happy, sometimes even joyful, full of hope, full of despair, realise some of our goals, fail in others, make and lose friends and those loved, and wonder: what is it all for, and where do we go from here?

There are many, I among them, who believe that in all the apparent confusion of our lives there is hope. Indeed hope is eternal because life is eternal. Hope is our guiding star: it is not mere surrender of thought or resignation of will; it is founded upon certainty since if that were not so there would long since have been an end to the human gift for enduring against all hardships.

Since hope is eternal, what else is eternal? We are eternal because we are spirit beings. I do not mean that we are as the traditional paintings and carvings of angels—pure, holy, calm beyond our knowing, engaged always in acts of worship, mercy or inspiration as though in their world there is no fear, no anger, no hate, only love, mercy—and no pain. Especially pain.

The pictured and carved angels appear to have all the qualities we admire but seldom find expressed in human beings like ourselves. We need not pause to speculate on angels but we may think about being eternal and trust that on the way to our development we may, in due time, express some of the qualities painted and carved by those men and women of inspiration, the artists. We are eternal and also are spirits, whether we choose angels as examples, or ourselves.

There has to be a reason why we are here. If that were not so I believe we would have long since gone the way of other species who could not survive the changing environments of nature. We persist in spite of our continuing problems—and crises. We survive and grow, inwardly, because of our trials. In dealing with our problems we develop our spirit natures because we have to achieve an evolution as continuous as life itself; evolution is the garment of continuous creation.

Why am I so confident? I have no special insight into the meaning of life. I have no authority from any source to tell anyone what to do with his or her life. I have some facts, many experiences and an urge to share them with anyone who will pay attention. My prophecies are easy to make because they arise from what has happened and what is happening continuously, beginning with the statement already made: we are spirits and are on the path by which we may, in immeasurable time, become spiritual, or spiritualised. How can such a statement be supported?

Few persons living today can say they have not heard of the concept of a life beyond death, irrespective of whether they believe or disbelieve that view. If there is no life after death I am a false prophet and must despair at having misled anyone. But I am sure of the ground because the evidence, day by day, year by year, century by century, age upon age proclaims what is said here. Since there is a life beyond death what are its implications? Since there is such a life, how do we inquire into it? That is not difficult. The means are available if we take the trouble to find them. In the seeking there will be difficulties. Such an adventure has its difficulties since the prize to be won is of inestimable value. Of course we will have difficulties; we have difficulties without moving from our chairs. That is our nature, in part. To begin such a search eventually, if we persist, will result in wisdom beyond the teachings of all the sages because we will be learning from life and what we learn will be permanent because we will be venturing into awareness of eternity.

Since there is a life in the Beyond and departed humans like ourselves live there and are fully occupied, are they any different from we who are still tenants of this world? They still are essentially as we are. To my certain knowledge they do not lose anything of their humanity nor of their desire to help others. We leave this place to become resident in our true homes, all, without exception, because we have no choice but to move forward in evolution.

It is a paradox to reflect that the great question confronting all of us: "If a man die, shall he live again?" should be so simply answered. The claim is made and proved that since many millions living on earth today have so much evidence of survival of bodily death, it may be said to be beyond discussion, except that we each seek our own verification of the facts as in all other important aspects of our lives.

Life now appears, in face of all that is claimed here, to be a cooperative venture in evolution with partners on both sides of the veil working together, without expectation of being recognised yet giving more than any hero, any warrior, indeed more than any other class of individual could give this world. It is a large claim. But when we are confronted with the consequences flowing from the discoveries cited, they must be accepted and sustained. There is no other teaching with such a power, with such impact yet it has to make its way into each soul's deepest recesses individually before the visible and tangible effects can be known.

It is easy to prophesy, without fear of failure, some of the changes which follow the discovery of the Life Continuous; rich in meaning and opportunity for all without exception, according to our capacity to take advantage of the many gains in knowledge which will be made available.

Prophecy is easy to make because the signs are

abundant, among them the evidence for Survival, and now the modern spirit healing mission, the greatest effort of its kind. That is my assessment alone and cannot be laid to anyone else. The modern healing mission is such an emerging force in society that it must touch all in time because we are all concerned with ourselves, naturally and properly, and we all desire to live free from bodily stress. In short, we seek maximum expression.

Although known in all times, spirit teaching within the past century, or even less, has pierced the outer defences of materialism, and has produced great changes in our thinking. Now comes the army of healers who by their benign service enlarge the gaps in those defences and so permit the liberating army to pour through. It has been a long and arduous struggle. But it will continue with increased force until we are again on the road to self-discovery supported by self-discipline, not of the penal kind but of the liberated heart and mind.

There must be a reason why spirit healing makes so much headway in Britain and so little elsewhere. In the past 50 years alone the healing movement has grown to such strength that it has touched all classes. By force of the pioneers, many unnamed, it has spread everywhere in Britain, without cathedrals, without ranks, without hierarchies, without creeds and dogmas and without taking tribute from those who are served.

The "large activity" already mentioned is called spirit healing because it is healing of the mind and spirit and body, by spirit people in cooperation with sensitive people on earth, who are trained how to serve following development of their potentials for the work. That is one aspect of self-discovery—that we may be so constituted as to act as conscious channels of spirit power, suitably modified, to achieve healing. Much, of course, has been written about self-discovery. This approach makes of the healing process a reality in the life of a person. Here, they may say, is something they can grasp mentally and here is a way they can serve which is not discoverable by any other means than self-development. That is the reason there are so many healers giving their time and devotion for the aid, comfort and healing of others.

Those who are trained how to cooperate are directed silently, as a rule, by spirits trained for their specific services. The healing is always cooperative although the healer on earth may not always be aware of the process. The forces, or energies, employed by the spirit healers in the beyond are, so far, beyond scientific recognition. The day will come when these forces or energies will be identified and employed more fully for human welfare. That is another prophecy.

This is not to say that all who seek spirit healing are immediately and wholly made well. This is not true of the sick who seek orthodox medical or surgical aid. Some bodily conditions are beyond remedy, such as wasted limbs and truly atrophied organs.

I am aware that many books have been written about spirit healing. There is much information about methods and sources of the power used—and much misinformation. There are schools of thought which prefer to refer its healing source to various religious leaders of the past and to them exclusively. These do not testify, although the healing goes on.

It could well be that all healing is part of a universal ministry and that even where the origin is debated by us on earth the healing goes on nevertheless. To lose time and opportunity in such controversy is unwise. That holds true, with this observation: that knowledge is always better than ignorance, even to stubborn ignorance in face of the facts. For, by becoming aware of those who direct their healing, the spirit healers in our midst acquire or develop a combination of resources and aptitudes that makes for more and more effective healing.

In the course of the long record of spirit healing much experience has been gathered on both sides of the veil. Each kind of healing has its advantages—and its limitations; there is no cure-all because we each have our own inheritance. We each arrive on earth with our individual matrix of merits and defects, all woven into the web of our potential. The former we have to increase, the latter we have to remedy, and we do so in the always changing stream of life. Our positive and negative characteristics are the battlegrounds of our development. The battles have their gains and losses also, and in the aftermath of our own internal conflicts we become aware of the yearning to help our fellows. What can we do when the struggle seems to be beyond us? Only the best we can with what we have in the conditions we are in. There is no magic, no miracle. We are, in a sense, our own creators. Since creation is an eternal drama, we always have time and opportunity to grow. To heal is to grow and to aid others in their growing.

There is a difference between being a spirit and being spiritual, lest you think these are interchangeable terms. We are of all kinds of spirits, at different stages of development. We are not instantly changed into angels the moment we are free from earth. If that were so, the whole healing mission would not be required. We are spirits because that is how we are created. We are spiritualised by our own efforts to become as they are whose entire being is closely attuned to spirit life and laws and conduct. We develop our spiritual natures by serving others and so come to the condition of attunement. Having shed the stains of earth we eventually become as they are who have reached higher in development than we may imagine on earth. Healing is one service by which we may raise our consciousness closer towards what it is destined to be.

To what do we aspire, since our goal cannot be wholly realised on earth; is it a temporary residence, a place for education? I believe we aspire toward becoming, in a conscious state, what we regard as being closest to our ideal of ourselves. It is a mature view to realise that an ideal is not an end in evolution but a way station. Therefore, men and women turn their thoughts towards development of those gifts which they all know are of the nature of the innate and the permanent; that is the spiritual gifts. Since these cannot be realised by self-service we tend, all of us, to turn towards others and ask what we may do for them.

The sum of this and other frustrations, the frustration of the expression of the soul fully, and our despair at finding our way is a major cause of the disharmony in this world and within our own natures. That disharmony long continued leads to disease since we are not then in harmony, at ease, within ourselves. This is not a new concept but it describes much thought. It is stimulating, to me, to think that in preparing to write this book I had the pleasure of discussions with the world's most eminent healer, Harry Edwards, in the course of which we talked much of that concept. I will try to bring out, later, my reasons for accepting that view, based upon the experiences of Edwards and others.

How may we become physicians of the soul, where the key to health is kept? That is what we also have to explore. On the way we will recognise that we carry our prospects and defects with us: that is why spirit teachers refer to our burdens and urge us to bear with one another as we carry our burdens towards that condition in evolution where we may lay them down for the last time since we will no longer require them.

In the spirit world, as here, excellence is a desirable

goal. Those who are healers there, together with doctors and scientists of all classes, do not abandon all they have learned because they have parted from their physical bodies. They continue their professions and extend their knowledge because the growing pool of experience is available to them and to those who went before them. What else would they do, since they are aware of the distress to be relieved on this planet? All their accumulated expertise and skill and knowledge is turned toward service, the only currency of the spirit. The spirit healers and scientists work with their methods of bridging the gap between our matter and their equivalent of matter. They say they have procedures not yet explicable to us since there are no common terms of reference. In time, the terms will be found. Their accumulated knowledge turns into greater capability. Experimentation is unending, as on earth. They, as we, each have their places in the grand scheme of eternal life. As we advance from grade to grade, as it were, by service rendered, the yearning grows to serve more and more.

If this is too idealistic a picture, it is a reasonable likeness of what we are told by those who report on life, and healing, from the spirit world. They should know.

How we become aware of our healing potential will be stated as well as the organised teaching to prepare emerging healers. Nothing is left to the hazards of uninformed experimentation.

Evidence for these statements is attested by thousands who have already joined the army of those who heal by the power of the spirit. There are many more armies to be recruited and trained and sent into the war on fear, ignorance, superstition—and disease.

HEALING

Continuous Life

Physical Evidence for Materialisation

Analysis of Ectoplasm

Personal Experiences

Communication with Spirits

States of Consciousness

The Spiritual Gifts

The Psychic Story of the Nazarene

Evolution of the Psychic Nature

A world in pain cries out for healing not of the body alone but from the stress of anguished minds. The void answers—Silence.

Our human world, filled with wonders and terrors, stumbles from one man-made crisis to another and seems, by its own record, to continue on its wild course, until some combination of crises overbears all human efforts to find solutions. We begin again the sorry climb back to our earned place in evolution. Once more we have added to our own burdens, defeated for a while by revolutions and other man-made upheavals because we have once again broken the laws of nature and of our spiritual nature.

This is no basis for shaping a prophecy of doom. The immediate causes and effects of our present condition are well known to the better-informed groups of mankind, whose hands and minds control the levers of power. These hands have but to reach out for a button in a crisis of despair and we will have taken the final step in a tragedy of universal proportions when the situation could so easily have been benign and kind to all mankind's welfare.

We are so many upon the earth. Our societies are now so complex. We have so many mouths to feed, so many undeveloped minds to nourish with knowledge, we have so many legacies of wrongdoing, in spite of our efforts, to improve the human lot that we cannot find a clear, unburdened starting place for the greater tasks we should be concerned with, day and night, year by year, century by century.

There is no continuity within and among the nations. Only one step has been taken to ensure that, by agreement, some of the nations, by majority vote, may talk together before they die together. The efforts of men to cooperate in some important situations, as in the case of the United Nations, show that there is, at this late date, a probability that we are learning, if not to live by love then by fear in a common danger and to work together if only for self-preservation.

The facts and opinion of that situation, important to every soul on earth, are not the burden of this story. My purpose is to tell a story of the Life Continuous, chiefly as it speaks to us of the psychic and spiritual nature of man and of what flows from knowledge and application of these facts and powers.

Much of the story is taken up with the healing of the spirit of man by the spirit of life, of the mind by the mind, of the psychic nature by the psychic nature; the nature and powers of these three aspects or gifts comprising the only holy trinity affecting mankind—the body, the psychic nature and the spiritual nature. That trinity does not demand worship, supplications, entreaties, penances or any other of the many acts considered essential to mankind if it is to find grace, if not favour with God.

I hold that knowledge of our true, therefore, threefold nature, is essential for us in our efforts at understanding ourselves and all others. That knowledge is essential if we are to understand how we are to work together. That knowledge should help us live without willing hurt to anyone so that we may move on in our evolution without the periodic crises that appear to have been mankind's greatest contribution to its own, universal, distress.

It is much too late in our evolution for us to arrive at such knowledge by hints, furtive telling of direct personal experiences and by all the indirections we practice upon one another.

My positions are taken openly and without fear that I will have to retrace my steps because a new set of facts has been uncovered to confound conviction and show that what is claimed to be true is something wholly different and for reasons other than those given here. It is now claimed that this case, this story, where it is built upon the foregoing foundation, is based upon phenomena observed, confirmed by repetition in like circumstances, that the events reported are not known by hint, roundabout explanations, unexamined faith, inferences, myths, symbols, folklore and tradition.

Among the phenomena observed, and much of it recorded, are the following:

Appearances in part and in full form of deceased persons so clearly that they are identified. These appearances called materialisations are produced by the moulding of ectoplasm, a substance extruded from the medium's body by spirit action. These materialisations, many of which have been photographed, cannot be caused by other than spirit intelligence.

The ectoplasm has been chemically analysed and is reported to be substantially albumen. Also the weight of the ectoplasm used in producing the likenesses of the deceased has been recorded in scientific experiments and is found to be within an ounce or two of the weight loss registered with the medium on a scale.

Materialised likenesses have been known to walk, dance, talk, sing—and engage in conversations in the course of which evidential statements as to identity and continued existence have been made. To the touch the materialised forms are humanly warm, as I can personally testify since I have been embraced and kissed by a relative who proved her survival to me in circumstances leaving no doubt as to the reality of the phenomenon.

Literature on the subject of physical phenomena produced by or through mediums is extensive but much neglected. Such mediumship is rarely available today, prompting the speculation that, perhaps, the energy used in that effort is now transferred to healing. That is my theory, since I hold that all phenomena moves in cycles as the energy is allocated and that we are now deeply committed to healing because of its relevance to the conditions in public thought developed by the massive effort proving Survival through message-bearing mediums. Even a slight acquaintance with the phenomena of materialisation will show how complex is the field.

I suggest that the reader ponder where and what is the intelligence that produces these remarkable manifestations. The role of the mind in this situation has to be examined. There is something in the foregoing for the open-minded physicist to ponder. There is also something in the following for the plain citizen to ponder:

What is the nature of the intelligence which produced the raps on the wooden walls of a rural cottage in Hydesville, New York, some 130 years ago and led to the development of the wide range of evidence in between that outpouring and the current and developing healing mission?

The phenomenon of delivering messages from the other world to their relatives and friends in this world through the gifts of clairvoyance, clairaudience and trance speaking is too well established to be contested. The case has been proved in every form of publication, including television. No records are kept of the totals of factual cases; they are too many. Such mediumship involves many of the conditions required in the development of healing: it is based upon cooperation between the two worlds.

The closer the cooperation and the more intimate the merging of the states of consciousness, the more productive the mediumship. The phenomenon of moving objects at a distance is akin to materialisation—the objects are moved by ectoplasmic rods and other structures, under intelligent direction. There is no other satisfactory explanation. That phenomenon is also well documented—and neglected by science.

Then there is a whole range of mental gifts manifest through what is miscalled automatic writing. There is nothing automatic about it. Automatic means mechanical. In this case there is nothing mechanical. The writers of such works are, of course, psychics and some of the better ones, mediums who act as cooperators in the communications from spirits.

The mind of the medium, or sensitive, if the word medium displeases, is influenced to write statements often of great beauty and appeal, teaching of an exalted nature and, in general, indicates that personalities other than the sensitive dominate the thought and the mode of its expression. The literature of this phenomenon is well worth the study of even the most sceptical of inquirers.

Writings of this kind have persuaded even theologians that they had witnessed the recording of statements which throw new light on areas of the Bible. Indeed, without such writings, I maintain, there would not be any Bible at all. And that same book is full of evidence of the kind we are discussing here.

I have witnessed spirit-inspired writing and can assert that because of the speed of dictation, without error or grammatical flaws, with a flowing syntax and import of the message received, it must have issued from a superior mind, superior to the medium's—and most of the observers', including mine.

I have also, as have others, experienced thought transference and the transmission of identical images between two cities about 200 miles apart—simultaneously. Given the premise of spirit minds working in cooperation with sensitives there is no logical objection to the claim. In like conditions I am confident others could have the experience repeated. The problem is to find the developed psychics or mediums to serve as catalysts.

In addition to the psychic phenomena witnessed by contempories, there is the evidence of one of the world's great scientists, Sir Alfred Russel Wallace, relating to his lifetime experience. The phenomena he lists in his book, *Miracles and Modern Spiritualism*, in two categories, the physical, in which material bodies are acted upon, or seeming material bodies are produced, and the mental, consisting of a display of powers or faculties not known in the medium's normal state.

*Physical:* Producing sounds of all kinds, from a delicate tick to heavy blows as from a hammer; altering the weight of bodies; movement of physical bodies without human contact or agency; raising bodies into the air; transporting bodies to a distance out of and into closed rooms; releasing mediums from every kind of bonds, even from welded iron rings.

*Chemical:* Preserving from the effects of fire, production of perfumes and an anaesthetic.

*Direct Writing and Drawing:* Producing writing or drawing on marked papers placed in such positions that neither hand nor foot can touch them; sometimes visibly to the spectators, a pencil rising up and writing or drawing apparently by itself; writing on enclosed slates.

*Musical:* Instruments of various kinds played without human agency, from a hand-bell to a closed piano; original compositions of a high order and, in current times, compositions in the manner of celebrated composers who appear to the mediums to dictate the scores, note by note, together with directions as to technique.

*Spirit Forms:* The whole range of recorded materialisations, from a hand to full, human-scale figures which move as do human beings in the flesh. These have been described elsewhere.

*Spirit Photographs:* In the case of the famous medium, John Myers, the percentage of recognised forms appearing on plates and film approached 80. There are scores of instances of spirit photography.

*Automatic Writing:* Sometimes in trance the medium writes involuntarily sometimes in a condition difficult to describe, often of subjects not premeditated, sometimes beyond normal capacity, sometimes in languages not known, sometimes in mirror script, sometimes conveying information and views contrary to the medium's. Works of high literary value have been obtained in this way.

*Clairvoyance, Clairaudience:* A whole range of phenomena is known under this heading, from the appearance of the deceased who give visual evidence of their identities along with statements of facts of a striking nature. Sometimes the clairaudience supports the clairvoyance. These two manifestations are observed most in public demonstrations.

*Trance Speaking:* This is analogous to automatic writing except that the changes in voice are additional evidence. Children as well as mature adults, with all ages between, have demonstrated this gift. One example is cited by a distinguished lawyer of another day. Serjeant Cox reports: "I have heard an uneducated barman, when in a state of trance, maintain a dialogue with a party of philosophers on 'Reason and Foreknowledge, Will and Fate' and hold his own against them. I have put to him the most difficult questions in psychology, and received answers, always thoughtful, often full of wisdom and invariably conveyed in choice and elegant language. Nevertheless, a quarter of an hour afterwards, when released from the trance, he would be unable to answer the simplest query on a philosophical subject, and was even at a loss for sufficient language to express a commonplace idea."

This is a familiar experience, to this day.

The now established supremacy of spirit healing was not so well known in that day, the day of the great researchers in the scientific field.

We have here opened up a series of thoughts and considerations that will in the not too distant future turn inquiring minds to study these things without prejudice. If we do not have greater knowledge of what we are, physically, psychically and spiritually, we will always be floundering in the unproved assertions of specialists who have kept the doors of their minds firmly bolted against the intrustion of aspects of truths about ourselves which rightfully should be available to all. This is not a rare occurrence in human history. We have only to stretch forth our hands to touch spirit reality.

What else could the spirit reformers do to persuade human minds that they are what they claim to be? What more is required—an unending flow of miracles until the miraculous becomes the commonplace and human caprice tires of more and more of the same? To dwell in a thought world of miracles every day is to abandon reason and the growth of our souls. The miraculous is the twin of the superstitious, everywhere and in all societies at all times.

We may, if we are attuned, draw from the endless ocean of thought all the inspiration we require, provided we also have undergone the self-discipline of education. This is not to say that the academic life is the only path to inspiration. Judged by the output of those who have produced the world's greatest thoughts, the case for intellectualism alone as a sure magnet for attracting new truths is not proved. Whether we are intellectually oriented or whether we have receptive—and attuned—

natures the advantage goes to the attuned for they are less biased in respect of the materialist approach.

The ocean of thought is available to all, directly according to the capacity to receive. It is a new concept that I argue here since those who approach the same situation from a different base of thought will always lose their way. Thought flows as does any liquid—according to the law of gravity, spiritual or material, whether the scientists say it is electro-magnetic, or something else. No man has yet charted the thought flow in which we all live. But it is there because what has been proved so far in this study cannot be laid aside. There is no area of human concern for the betterment, or improvement, of the human condition where the spirit healing, teaching and inspiration are absent. The degree to which it becomes effective depends mostly upon us, for the many healers, teachers and inspirers are available on the other side of the veil—but not yet in sufficient quantity, and quality, on our side.

Most of the persons in the named categories come from those who seek development in the Spiritualist movement. It needs not be so exclusively for the healing power is available on the same terms and conditions—everywhere and to all. Where the servers make themselves available the healing will begin, little by little.

So, we begin with the phenomena to attract the attention of those who incline in the healing direction until they reach clearer views and more substantial knowledge of what we are. Then they can begin to cooperate with those other women and men, brothers and sisters if you like, who have passed through this world and are so eager to cooperate with us in the common enterprise of achieving what we have to become—spiritualised citizens in this world.

In attempting to cover the entire case for the existence and manifestation of the spirit world I have already outlined some of the better known phenomena. From the period beginning about 130 years ago—the advent of the Spiritualist movement—the evidence has continued. Just when some sceptics asserted that it was a movement without a future—or had surges of interest based upon widespread griefs caused by wars—the evidence increased until it reached the proportions described.

The case for the phenomena is unassailable. The case for the vast increase in healing is also unassailable—if we take rational standards for our assessments. The statistics alone are overwhelming—some 15 million requests alone to one healer, Harry Edwards, in the course of his more than 40 years of service. It appears now that, having broken the barriers of resistance to evidence of Survival, the directing organisation in the spirit world increased its healing mission.

To show there is a direct link between the psychic events of biblical times, statements from the testaments alone should suffice. To show that there is a direct link from ancient times to the present science of spirit healing it is only necessary to place current healing and biblical healing alongside one another. If they match in all major respects then the case for their identical origins is proved. My convictions on these points may not be persuasive at all points, so it is in order to attempt analysis of selected events to establish common effects arising from common causes.

What did happen in the Holy Land that is so important to this aspect of the case for Man the Healer? If we take the Old Testament as a record it is not as clear to the phenomena of healing as it is for other, physical phenomena. The Old Testament is a compilation of the events in several cultures which had sufficient commonality with events in Israel that they were edited into one, somewhat disjointed narrative. But, in the case of the New Testament there was sufficient phenomena of several kinds to enable a more or less coherent statement to be made since the events occurred in only one culture in a limited period and area. This is not discounted by the fact that the basic gospel writing has internal contradiction of fact; the healing is sequential, reported in detail and frank as to circumstances, as any thoughtful person may discover in a point by point comparison. What does emerge is that many were healed, mainly by the Nazarene, in public, some in his presence, even in the press of crowds, some at a distance and in all a most impressive record.

This is, in no way, different from the improved healing science of today: large numbers attend healing demonstrations and witness cures and improvements in all manner of diseases treated. Modern healings are more numerous because we have larger populations, travel is easy and communications are at our fingertips. One factor stands out in the comparison as between ancient and modern healing—healing at a distance. The healing in the Bible of the Roman centurion's servant, upon his request, is a classic since it set the test of the claim that healing energies are transmitted through space to the recipient and that cures result.

In modern healing tens of thousands of persons have been so cured. The evidence is overwhelming that this is the case. It is mainly in the healing that the phenomena of the Bible time is repeated; the other aspects of phenomena are singular, for the most part, since they are not repeated. It may be that the scribes confined themselves to healing because they had an exciting story to tell of the seemingly miraculous. Modern demonstrations are infinitely repeatable; miracles are one of a kind. Does this mean we have to become more spiritual or that the knowledge of nature's finer forces is increasing on both sides of the veil, and for other reasons to be stated?

An example: the dividing of the Red Sea by Moses is singular. The Mosaic plagues upon Egypt is a singular incident. Daniel in the lions' den has not been repeated, neither was the writing on the wall that so startled Nebuchadnezzar. Moses appears to have been one of the most remarkable of mediums; his being discovered by a princess in the bulrushes, his receiving the commandments, his guiding the Israelites out of Egypt and finally his appearance after death with Elija to encourage the Nazarene to persist in his mission although they said he "would accomplish his decease in Jerusalem". These are non-repeatable events, not miracles, but psychic phenomena.

It is not to be forgotten that while the spirit return of Jesus is held to be a singular, one-time miracle, the spirit return of Moses and Elija cannot be dismissed.

It may be that other like events did occur and that records of them are secreted in some Arabian shepherd's cave, sealed in jars, awaiting a favourable upturn in the market for such items. This has happened in our times. On one side, the case is made for a common pattern of events, or phenomena, occurring on the initiative of spirit people to attract the attention of earth people to some of the basic facts of life—and evolution.

To tell the Nazarene story in summary: this wonderful spirit was chosen by his brotherhood in the spirit to serve as their medium on earth during a period not unlike the present in some essentials. Empires had fallen, nations were in turmoil, ignorance was the normal condition. The nation into which the Nazarene was born was still under Roman rule. Rome itself was undergoing vast changes which affected the western world. How better to draw man's attention to the psychic and the spiritual than by popular demonstration?

This was done, dramatically, ending or seeming to end, with a tragedy that turned into a triumph when the

Nazarene kept his promise to return from the tomb. From that point human history changed because his medium, Paul, and the other disciples carried his teaching and some psychic demonstrations throughout the known world. The Greek and Hebrew cultures mingled. Plato and Paul became the guiding minds. The rest is history, not always accurately told.

How did the Nazarene impress his listeners? He taught in parables, in folk language, not as we moderns do with many words that tend to confuse. He illustrated his teaching with healing and with the power of his personality, although we do not have any record to describe him. The imaginative likenesses of him were made much later to establish stereotypes.

If you will receive this statement it may explain something: from the spirit world it is said that the Nazarene inspires much that is done in the mission today to enlighten man as to his true nature so that he may realise himself and live and develop as he is intended to do. It is also said that he is an advanced soul perhaps the most advanced to have walked this earth.

This aspect is not essential to an exposition of the healing mission but I am often asked about it and have set it down.

Now that we have left the world of miracles, we must examine what happened to the healing mission in the interval between the deaths of the Nazarene's disciples, through the acceptance of the Christian church as a state-favoured group. The consequences of that political manoeuvre are with us still for they include the long, dank, desperate Dark Age, when the human mind—and the human spirit—were suppressed. The darkness was relieved here and there by the visions of lonely mystics, men and women, sensitive to the spirit.

The influence of the Renaissance enabled men to rise from their knees to walk in the sunlight of awareness

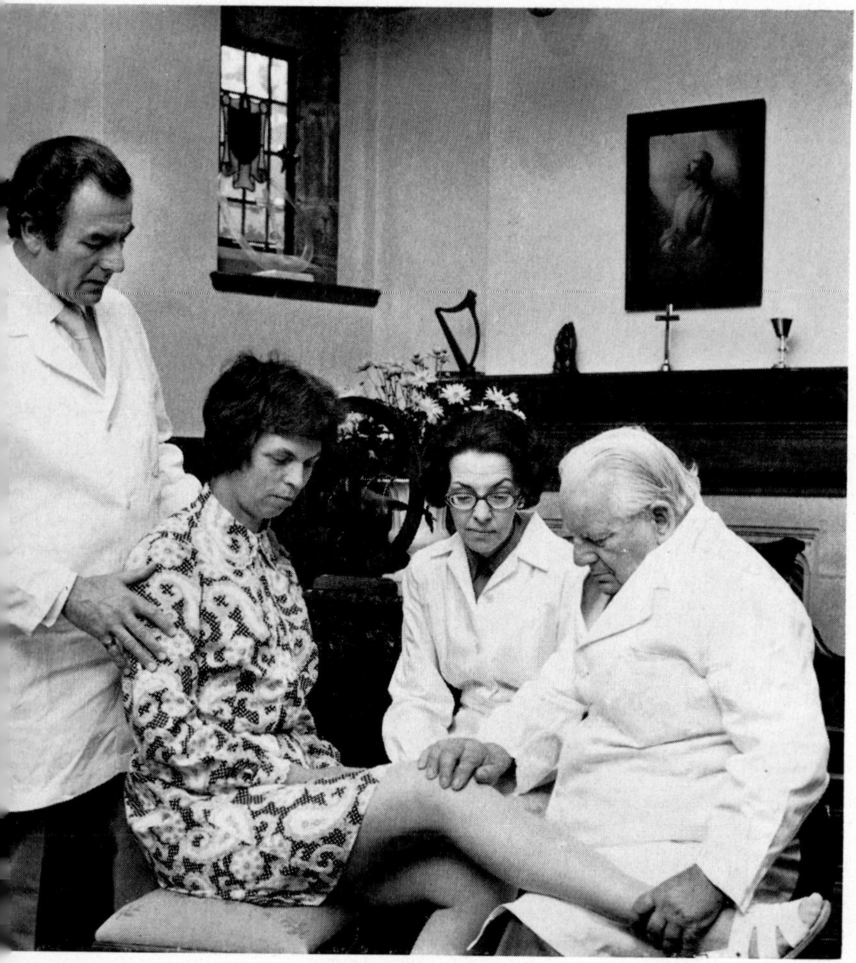

HEALING IN THE SANCTUARY

Harry Edwards, with his colleagues Ray and Joan Branch, healing in his world-renowned Spiritual Healing Sanctuary at Shere, near Guildford, Surrey.

HARRY EDWARDS
seen here giving healing at the Royal Albert Hall in London, before a capacity audience of 5,000.

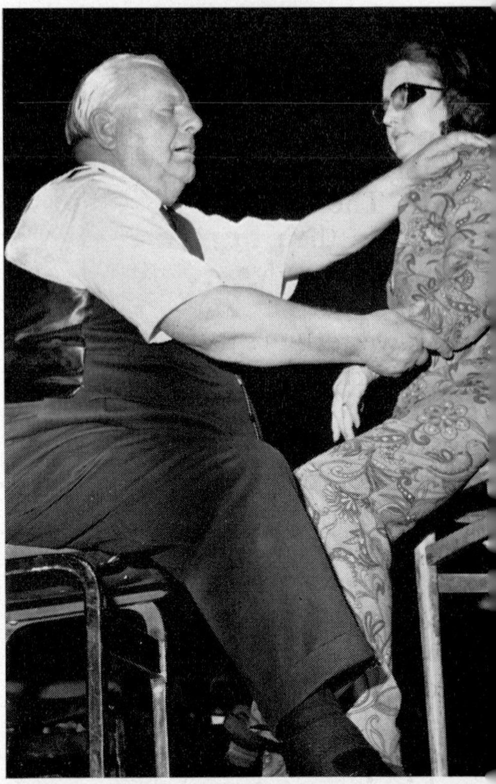

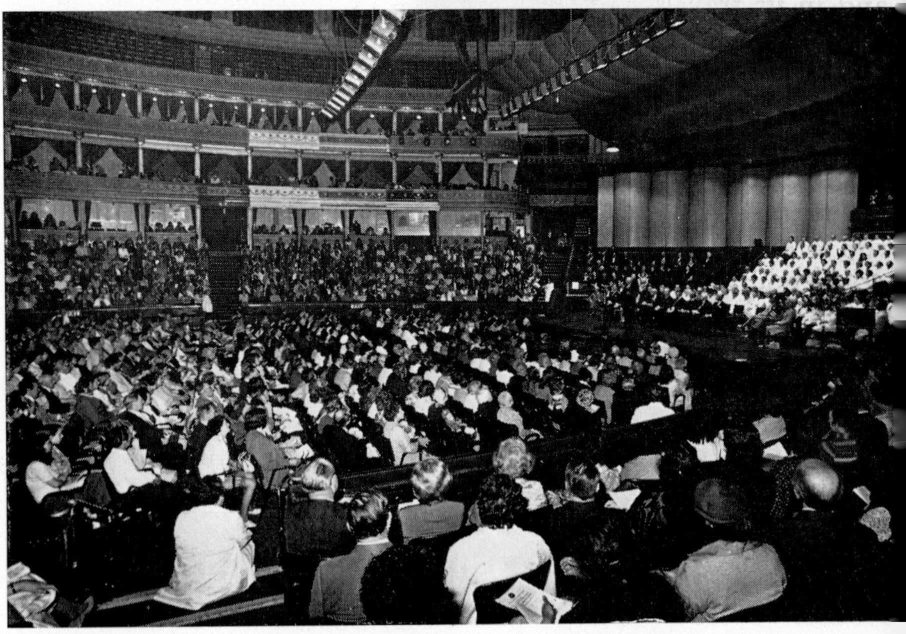

Part of the vast congregation at the Royal Albert Hall

that power is not all and that there is more to mankind than flesh. The Dark Night of the human soul was ending. Even within the state church there was ferment. The dissidents formed their own organisations which, in their turn, attempted the continuing censorship of knowledge.

The spirit persisted and registered a notable victory when western man imitated the Chinese and brought the art of printing to the relief of mankind. That was a great day. Men could then speak to one another at a distance through a little ink and some symbols on paper. This is not to say that there were no records before then. There were, but they were not available in quantity so that men could study and compare—and improve what was written.

England had the distinction of liberating the Bible from its Latin prison. England struck off the chains which held the Bible bound to the altar under the watchful eye of the priest. The world had changed. The world mind, in the west, was on its way to a great adventure and in its travels had to be made aware once more of the truths of its spiritual origin and its psychic gifts.

In the centuries between the end of the Nazarene's visit and the proliferation of printing the human mind had made advances and was ready to exploit its knowledge of physical nature, leading to science, which led to technologies that altered the landscapes and in the long run brought man, once again, to consideration of his origin and destiny since he had discovered a power with which he could destroy his planet.

It is at that point that spirit evidence of human survival of death reached a peak. The healing gift was also developing, held in check only until the mind was fertilised by the evidence for Survival.

Modern healing had its forerunner in the mesmerists, the hypnotists, the homeopaths and in plain healers like the Wesley brothers, the Quakers and many others. But it is the distinction of the Spiritualists that they made most impact. Their achievement in demonstration won the confirmation of eminent scientists, writers, statesmen—and of millions of citizens who were ready to know what had long been promised.

Since the human mind had become accustomed to reading this increased the mind's capacity to receive thoughts. People of the Nazarene's time or in Plato's Greece could not absorb, say, the concepts of modern chemistry, travel, communication, sheer speed, rapidity of physical movement, clashes of opinion—and of the kinds of wars we managed to arrange without consent of the intended victims.

Religions have been changed by thought alone, men have taken off into space by thought alone, men know how to communicate by bouncing a message from a satellite in the sky, by thought alone. Living conditions have improved—and, also, disease in wide areas has also increased. We have so much more and so much less. We may have all we desire physically. Yet the minds of men and women are afraid. And they still cry out in pain.

Most of us now accept that mankind is resigned to living by crises because it does not know of a better way or has given up thinking beyond the immediate future. How do we find a remedy for what ails us? There are no remedies for earthquakes, nor, so far for nuclear weapons, except more and more destructive nuclear weapons. It is a wry commentary that, having come close to nature's own powers, we are afraid of the consequences of using them in war. If there is any concept of an escape, or a remedy, it has not yet been published although many powerful intellects have been and are at work on such questions.

Let us begin with the view, or teaching (which it is) that man is a trinity, the only holy trinity, of body, psychic nature and spirit (or soul). The effects of the expressions of that trinity have been described variously in the preceding accounts of psychic phenomena, ancient and modern. Where do we now find evidence for the existence and use of the powers expressed through our threefold nature? By what phenomena may these be recognised?

Any tourist in a hurried visit to a strange land may find the ruins of great empires and civilisations. That is some evidence that the empires and civilisations existed. What of the citizens who once walked the broken streets? Are they no more, in any way? Or, do they have another state of existence? Is there something beyond the Something of existence upon earth?

The silent stones stand witness mute to the departed glory of massive anonymity, to departed treachery or infamy. Here and there are shards, bits of columns, an inscription or two, something for a museum, nothing for life. Other records may be found more or less intact, a manuscript, household implements, a trinket or so. This, to experts, may tell much of the things. What of the citizens who once lived here? Where have they gone? From nothing we came, to nothing we go? It is not credible that such effort should have no consequences. Is there another answer to our becoming the Impossible Nothing? I am sure there is. The next question is: how do we know?

Let us leave writing of history to historians. They write and re-write endlessly. Not one of them has written the history of women and men as spirit beings. Perhaps they do not know or do not care. Other projects may be more interesting.

There is no question that we dwell in a time of crisis, or in a series of crises. The world is a melting pot. This story is intended to make some contribution to the thinking of all who care to read it, since the notion of spirit influence upon human affairs is strange to many: to those who are aware of it there is no greater solace and encouragement than to persist in what we have discovered to be true.

To say that there is spirit influence in all our lives is not to state divine or saintly intervention in all of our daily affairs. Nor is it a placebo for troubles we bring upon ourselves. This story does state the case for the existence of spirit beings who employ spirit energies for the benefit of earth people. Such influence is not to be confused with the superstitions of the many who cannot trust either their own judgments or their innate capacity to deal with their own problems.

It does not argue for a life of endless prayer where a little direct, positive remedial action by us would meet the situation. Nothing in the case for spirit influence detracts from our imperative duty to deal with our own lives as best we can and when there appears not to be any hope to seek, silently, in the quiet of our own souls the answers to our questions.

We are not puppets made to dance and jerk upon a string in the hands of the master puppeteer without power of will to direct within limits of free will our own lives.

The case for spirit influence is found most evidentially in the services rendered by mediums and others who cooperate with such beings for the good and welfare of all of us, as we seek their counsel and aid.

In providing evidence of Survival, without mediums it could not be done. Why? Because we, at this stage of human development, are unable to raise our own consciousness to that level at which we can talk, face to face, with spirit people. If there is another way to gather experience of the spirit it is not commonly known. Even in those cases in which some claim they do talk, by themselves with the dead, they are their own mediums.

It is then a short step to saying that in due course mediumship is a natural gift, closer to the surface of consciousness in some than in others. This is also true of other gifts, else we would all be as eminent as the great ones in all of life's arts.

To become aware of our psychic natures requires only that we consider the situation calmly, without unprovable notions of evil spirits and the rest of the superstitions that abound today more than in less enlightened times. Let us all reflect calmly on the origin of our thoughts. If we are sufficiently self-disciplined we will quickly realise that our thoughts jump all over the place. Buddhists liken the mind to a monkey jumping on our hands, always in motion, without direction, until disciplined and taught what to do.

In that process of examining how we think we discover how to think our problems through—until our emotions take a hand in the process.

Then, having reached some measure of control over our thoughts, without any kind of ceremonial or other external apparatus of incantations, we may then direct them to a specific goal. It is a difficult exercise, without question, and here it may be helpful to retell an anecdote credited to Gautama Buddha: He came across an aged yogi on a river bank; with his disciples, the Buddha stopped, paid his respects to the old man and asked him what was the purpose of his meditations. The yogi said he had striven many years to be able to levitate himself across the river. Said Buddha, "If you give the boatman a few pennies he will row you across and save much time."

That may not be a true story, or anecdote, but it makes the point that we should get on with our lives as best we can with what we have at our disposal. The old yogi apparently did not have the psychic power of self-levitation, or maybe he did not know how it was done.

Since we each have a psychic nature we will find, in time, that by paying attention to it we become aware of thoughts we did not think for ourselves and of emotions that arise seemingly of themselves. We will also find that as we reflect or meditate new thoughts will arise unbidden into the mind. That is so simple that perhaps it should not be written because we humans do not, as a rule, like simple answers to simple questions.

Having outlined a theory of discovering our own psychic natures, how does it help in explaining spirit influence upon us? By the method just outlined.

My explanation is this: when we begin to discipline and explore our thoughts with the intention of having our psychic natures attuned to the point at which we become aware of spirit responses, we may decide we will try to become healers.

We may begin to feel we are aware of influences unnoticed before. That is how, in essence, our potential begins to make itself known to us. This, and the compassionate desire to help others, attracts those in the spirit who are in tune with our aspirations. I am persuaded they largely, silently and as a planned activity, make the first contact which becomes our awareness as we seek attunement towards healership.

As we persist in our thought control and development without tension or making a stern rule of concentration (which is self-defeating of our purpose), we become, gently, almost imperceptibly more and more aware of the spirit influence.

This is no claim that we should abandon reason as our guide; what fails to meet the test of our reason should be laid aside, or discarded. Frequently what is not acceptable as a guide at one point in our development will become clearer, later. We are discussing growth, not revelation of instant healership.

As our thoughts expand, we will realise the responsibilities of becoming a healer, an instrument for transmitting healing energy through our natures from the spirit world to someone close, or at a distance. You may see now that healing is a form of mediumship with the same kind of discipline as in other forms. Mediumship at its best approaches the pinnacle of human activity for the impact of its actions goes to the soul of the healer and to the recipient of healing, since it is in the soul that our own gifts have their being. And, it is in the soul that all spirit healing begins.

As we become more attuned to the source of healing power, we come to know more readily the intent of the spirit healers. Cooperation increases with increase of awareness which produces greater effectiveness.

What we do as mediums, healers or sensitives has influence not only on those healed but on others as they spread the word of their experiences. What greater testimony is there to healing than the very presence of the one healed?

These views of the influence of spirits upon physical life were, in the form stated here, not possible in other centuries because the human mind could not grasp them; there was no line of development—and there was a strict censorship on the teaching and writing on such matters; only the priests could deal with such matters, as they chose. Men's mouths were closed by flames; women were burned or done to death in other ways because they were psychics—and just women.

Thanks to the non-priestly discoveries of the printers, the scientists and the courageous men and women who would not give in, we arrived at mass communication between us in this world and, in time, at much increased communication between the two worlds.

It is significant that both kinds of communications developed in the same period.

It is clear that among the aims of those who direct the

spirit mission is reconciliation of the two worlds so that we will learn, slowly, the art of spiritual regeneration and, one by one, lay the foundations for a better, spiritualised mankind in which disease will be a rare exception.

This is a large claim. The ideas and claims are not all mine; only the presentation of them. You will choose what you will. Time and experience alone will decide.

Since this is a personal statement, maybe accounts of direct personal experiences in healing will be helpful in weighing this presentation. If a man claims to know something of a subject it is well that he should speak from his knowledge.

My first psychic experience goes back more than 40 years when one of my children, born with a hernia, was healed through the advice of a medium in Blackpool, England. She had the gift of reading letters in women's closed handbags, although she was scarcely literate. My wife and I had not met the medium till we attended one of her meetings. In addition to advice on the child's hernia, for which surgery had been discussed with a doctor, the medium suggested we change the child's diet, which had nothing to do with the hernia. He was a reluctant eater. We followed her simple advice. The child responded eagerly. The hernia healed without surgery.

Much later in London we became rich in experience of psychic phenomena; the other riches were harder to find.

Through careless treatment by a dentist, my wife had to be treated by a dental specialist. At a seance in our home, among many other items of evidence provided in controlled conditions, my wife received, on a piece of photographic paper, inside an envelope held in her hand, this message: "Watch for Good Friday". The message was in bold type. The medium was John Myers, a famous psychic photographer and healer.

My wife's pain increased in the brief period between the seance and that Good Friday. Early on Good Friday morning she was in such distress that I tried to reach the specialist who was treating her. He was out of town. I could not find a substitute. I tried to reach John Myers. He was, I was told, on his way to a luncheon engagement and had with him a visiting Indian psychic researcher. Silently, I called on Myers' guide, whom we knew well, and appealed for help. Not long afterwards Myers was on my doorstep, saying his guide had told him to come to our home to help my wife.

The Indian researcher informed me that Myers had changed direction so abruptly that he was almost involved in an accident.

Myers was entranced, my wife was put to sleep by the spirit guide . . . and there was a strong odour of a chemical in the room which I took to be ether. I have never had ether in my home.

The spirit guide talked with me on personal matters while, as he said, the spirit doctors were at work. He assured me that when my wife awakened the pain would be gone, and would not return. That was a promise. As soon as my wife awakened she clapped a hand to her mouth, exclaiming: "My God, the pain's gone." Sometime later while she was preparing rice for a meal she tasted a grain. The pain returned. As she reports: just as immediately a large black hand passed through her head and the pain ended.

I reported this happening to the dental specialist when my wife returned for treatment. He said only spirit healing could explain the healing.

Some years later, while I was orating on Spiritualism in Hyde Park, London, as I was nearing my peroration I noticed the dental specialist in the (small) crowd. He heard me as I said: "There is the doctor who can testify to what I have just said." He said nothing. He walked away. So did I. It was my farewell appearance after what was probably the shortest oratorical career at Hyde Park speakers' corner.

Later in London, during World War II, I became seriously ill with a high fever, as a result, I believe, of overwork. I overheard the doctor tell my wife that he could not do more for me—it was between God and myself. My wife then called Billy Parish, a famous spirit healer and close friend. He said he could not obtain transport quickly but would treat by absent healing, of which he was a pioneer, as I know from close personal investigation.

In my distress I felt as though two, large, silver-white hands touched the nape of my neck where the pain was most intense. I fell deeply asleep for some hours and, awakening, asked my wife to call Maurice Barbanell, editor of *Psychic News*, to come over to discuss a libel action in which we were then involved, one of the many exciting episodes in our long association in the Spiritualist movement.

Parish did not have to visit me in my home.

Some time later, a family friend and neighbour, member of a well-known Quaker family, told me her husband was seriously ill with cancer. She asked for spirit healing for him.

I called Parish who asked me to try to give healing while he sought transportation for the long trip from his East Sheen home. I did not think I could heal and did the usual things I had seen others doing, including laying on hands and concentrating. I learned later that concentration has nothing to do with healing.

Our neighbour died. His widow said later that the doctor said her husband was cured of cancer before his death. I cannot explain that. Some 30 years later we visited the widow in her home in England. A healing group meets there, as they now do in many homes all over Britain. In a quiet period she told me that my wife and I had removed her fear of death. She now helps others reach such growth.

In the course of my first visit to the United States I met, under my pen name, a medium from Columbus, Ohio. I say that because no one in that place where I saw her, Anderson, Indiana, knew me. Through her mediumship I talked with a sister I had not even known; she told me she had died at birth but that the children who came after her had not been told. She urged me to tell another sister, whom she correctly named, who lived in San Diego, California. I had no intention of ever visiting San Diego.

Then a materialised figure, saying she was a deceased aunt, greeted me, named herself correctly and to quieten my doubts showed me her very long, blonde hair. As a child, I, with others, used to ask her to sing for us and show us that her hair was so long she could sit on it. She turned to show me her long hair then asked me to walk to the far end of a long room with her. Because I was suffering from vaccinosis—in a heat wave—she touched my aching arm lightly. We talked on the slow walk and at parting she asked me to kiss her. I did so, dutifully. She laughed, saying I could do better than that. I did better. It was a warm woman I embraced.

That evening, still not known to anyone except an associate, we attended another seance at the same place. My aunt materialised again, greeted me and stepped aside to allow a young girl, materialised, to glide past me. She sat at a piano and asked what music I preferred. The phrase, Handel's Largo, came into my mind (I am not musical). The girl said it was not easy to do that on the piano and asked me to try something else. Immediately she began to play a Scottish air, "Will Ye No Come Back Again", and my aunt, long deceased, in a good voice sang it as only a Scotswoman could, accent of

Fifeshire and all. Then she vanished. Largo? That is the village in which she lived.

I told my sister in San Diego some time later of the seance. She wept with joy because, she said, it was true. She confirmed the statement by the first spirit to materialise that her name was Sarah, which I had been given by several mediums in London but which I could not place. The only person who knew was my sister in San Diego. My mother had died many years before I visited the United States.

These experiences do not make me an authority but, I believe, they qualify me as a man of some experience. They are a fraction of the whole. I believe that these, and many other experiences, were training for the work I do. The evidence was always there. I have never had to go seeking it, no matter where I was.

While much has been said about psychic matters in the past 130 years, or so, as an aside I can report taking part in what is called the healing of obsession, which is also miscalled possession. The first, obsession, is obstruction of another person, on earth, by a social misfit from this world still not rehabilitated in the other world. The second is the association of a benign and cooperative spirit with us. Ignorance makes the two identical, adds to the error the terrors of superstition. Priests and other meddlers become involved, Latin phrases are read and so on, and the vulgarisation reaches its peak hysteria when turned to profit.

In the cases of my experience, all that was required, with the aid of a medium, was to encourage the lost soul, to discuss his problems, to persuade him he was deceased and to urge him to look around for someone to enlighten him. This done, the obsession stops. The cause is in the unripe soul, projected into a world he does not know about, with his desires intact and his inability to function a source of anger and even vengeance. The true cause is society's for providing the conditions in which obsession's seeds are sown here and ripened there.

I quote some of my experiences to indicate we have a long way to go before we develop the society in which that particular disease will not occur.

# SCIENCE

Evidence of Life Beyond
Points Way to
Spirit Healing

Without Survival No
Spirit Healing

Faith Alone Does Not
Explain Healing

Healing at a Distance

Consciousness of Cells

15 Million Healings
by Edwards

Darwin and Russel Wallace;
from Scientific Theory to
Spiritualist Proof

Mind and Brain are
Different

## THE TRUE METAPHYSICAL

Since speculation may be defined as an idea waiting to be born in the mind we should examine some of the speculations of orthodox scientists on the prospects of their entering the next stage of inquiry and discovery beyond the physical: the metaphysical, the true metaphysical.

As this is the story of the origin and development of spirit healing, and of much springing from it, if we neglect the position of physical science the account will be incomplete. Scientists also try to peer through the mists into the future in its state of becoming. There are many who brush aside the idea that we can, in some conditions, become aware of the future because we know much that has happened and we know what is occurring now. Physical scientists sail in the same evolutionary ship as the spirit healers. The physicists especially are always on the lookout for what is to come, since they know that they are nearing the end of discovery in matter: they are hovering on the brink of what is in the becoming beyond this earthly realm. The prospect is revolutionary.

We who have some experience of that further state welcome any inquiry into the condition beyond the physical—again, the true metaphysical, the state beyond matter. We are persuaded that experience of spirit healing has provided us with insight into the other state and we are ready to share that experience because we believe it is beneficial to all souls. Our approach is as scientific as such an approach can be. We have uncovered powers not normally understood. These powers are proved by their effects. By their application to physical, mental and emotional ills their remedial nature is known. Our laboratory is the human race; or such portion of it that seeks our services.

This is not to develop a mystery. What is known by experience and knowledge derived from study, what is regularly demonstrated, what is repeated, what is subject to analysis, statistical and otherwise surely cannot be labelled mysterious. The position is this: we say, even assert, that because there is a life beyond physical death, human beings must live there in some state of consciousness. This is proved every day. The mass of evidence is now so great it may fairly be called overwhelmingly favourable. The concept has lodged in the western mind especially, and in Britain particularly. Briefly, the scientific position is that the case is not yet proved, even though the physical evidence should persuade any fair and open-minded person. This position is not to be argued all over again—after more than 130 years of demonstration.

Having established a concept in the thinking of at least one entire nation, Britain, the next step is healing, healing through men and women here on this earth. Now healing apart from medical treatment is not new to the human race. The records of all cultures bear testimony to its reality. Why, then, describe it now as part of a spirit-led mission to benefit all mankind? The answer is that, since there have been many changes in human affairs, and since much harm has been done by those who try to dominate human thought, the knowledge and practice of healing had been almost destroyed.

It became necessary to revive the knowledge, just as in the Western Renaissance it became essential to revive the spirit of inquiry. The human spirit has to be free; that is its destiny. To be free it has to know. It cannot know certain truths save by personal conviction, through the one-by-one method. One of the truths humanity had to re-learn was survival of human personality after bodily death. From that effort, which cost dear in suffering for those who pioneered it, came the current state of awareness of Survival, to capsulate a world of knowledge.

Once Survival was lodged in the human mind, there came the next step—its deepening. This is seen in the literature of communication between citizens of the earth and citizens of the spirit world. No thunder of mockery nor lightning of scorn, no fires, nor swords, nor persecutions, nor prisons will destroy that again. It is here, permanent, and will grow until we achieve our destiny as spirits with infinite capability.

Survival, being so established as an idea, how next do we serve the human soul? By his mind alone? He is resistant to all ideas not immediately useful to him in his need for security, continuance, comfort and satisfaction. Death is in his life; he labours more in faith of better things to come than in sure knowledge that they will come, if not now, tomorrow; if not tomorrow then another day, and as he nears the end of one journey he wonders, neither afraid nor confident, about what is to come after all, whether it is to be nothing and the darkness of unending night or a brighter day of birth in a promised land.

Is it so small a service to have rendered in lifting the burden of fear of death from the minds of millions? And, having done so, having beneficially changed much of human thought, should we then rest from our mission and cry "enough"? By experience we learn that we may not decide: we may cooperate or resist; with us, the plan will unfold, and if we withdraw, it will continue to unfold with others.

We have moved from providing evidence of Survival as our principal activity to the development of healing as an equal service which will, in time, further change and increase human though. The facts of spirit healing are impressive; the implications more so, for they open doors in minds shut tight for centuries against the entrance of concepts intended for our liberation.

Having proved so often that healing is done by the action of spirit beings on their human colleagues, we believe that scientists may learn much since they are regarded as the keepers of knowledge by a vast public, especially medical men because their principal concern is the body. What affects the body is a concern so deep that the appearance of any ill becomes a cause of profound concern.

Whether the medical world has done or is doing all that is required of it is another concern. The cost in money alone of maintaining health to some degree is a world question, therefore, any teaching and practice of any kind of healing, orthodox or unorthodox, must be considered carefully.

The attitude of physical scientists towards spirit healing is not commendable. They, not surprisingly, take the position that the very phrase, spirit healing, is a misnomer because they do not accept the proven fact—that there are spirit beings, intelligent, benign, resourceful, possessing knowledge they would share with us when we provide the conditions appropriate for communication between their world and ours. Since we are forced to begin with a breach in our communication with scientists, the problem of providing evidence suitable to their terms remains.

Individual medical men and scientists have joined our ranks at the risk of loss of standing and even of professional security. This should not be since we heal, not hurt, and we heal where the accepted, official healing arts fail.

When we succeed where other methods fail we are told it is all a matter of faith, or of "spontaneous remission", words to bridge gaps that cannot be bridged merely by language. What in this world is spontaneous when the sun rises and sets by order?

If faith alone is the cause of spirit healing, why include the spirit factor? If faith alone is the cause of cure why does not faith deliver cures for medical science? Does faith weaken when science intervenes? What is this magical faith? Is it belief without knowledge and if so, on whose part, the doctor's or the patient's, or the patient's family? Is faith a thing or a force, a kind of electro-magnetic energy? If the last mentioned then it should have been discovered by scientific methods. Imagine the effect of a scientifically proved energy called faith being applied in hospitals in our country alone! Think of the changes that would generate in society. No, the faith alone attitude will not explain what happens in spirit healing.

To say that faith alone is not the cause of cure is not to say faith has no place; it most certainly has, but it should be in league with knowledge. This removes spirit healing from the category of happenstance, chance, mystery, creed and fear and places it where it belongs—among the essential human sciences still not explained by any scientific or other theory.

In summary, St. Paul gave sound advice when he is reported to have counselled: faith is the substance of things hoped for, the evidence of things unseen. That is the conviction of a mystic who was also a healer, a medium. His reported experiences confirm that view. What is the substance he speaks of? What is the unseen he speaks of? If ever a prophet spoke of what is to come, it was Paul in that one utterance.

But, leaving Paul on one side, his position is that of spirit healers: to your faith add knowledge. Then the prophet gave a category of spiritual gifts. The category is the same today. The Pauline utterance in the spiritual field is as a signpost to us, if we but knew how to read it. After nearly 2,000 years his prophecy is verified in the healing being done today. In that sense science was anticipated and today scientists are slowly, very slowly moving toward confirming what was said in that ancient time and what is being demonstrated today. Spirit healing cannot be ignored because it is the way of the future.

Before we leave the faith-alone position, consider: Faith alone cannot explain the following healing:

Where the patient was unaware of a request for healing;

Where the patient was too young to know about faith, as in an infant or a child;

Where healing was sought by a friend or relative without the patient's knowledge;

Where the patient opposed the very idea of faith;

Where the patient was not in a condition to be told about healing and, most important, where the patient was healed at a distance merely on the basis of a written request to the healer by someone interested in the case.

If distant healing, it is argued, is another case of so-called spontaneous remission or is attributed to any cause but spirit healing, how do we account for the hundreds of thousands of distant healings? Has nature taken leave of her laws? Is there anarchy in heaven, is magic running wild, are all the healed persons untruthful when they report cures?

Science has an impossible task if it cares to refute our claims: it has another response—silence, and goes on with its established views while new truths make their channels in the human mind.

There is no method yet devised by man that will

prevent the eventual emergence of ideas. Scientists should have learned that from the tangled history of progress in science.

In addition to providing proof of survival of human personality beyond bodily death, Spiritualism, the principal factor in developing healers, provides a basis for all religions to regain much of the support they have lost by refusing to live according to the convictions of their founders. For, if a religion does not prove life beyond the grave, it is no longer religion. The rest, apart from healing, can be found in any one of many philosophies and, in some cases, nobler concepts of the art of living in human societies. We are the only ones who say yes to the historical question and prove it: "If a man die shall he live again?" Equally we answer yes to the question: if a man heals shall he heal again? Both are certain in a world of uncertainty.

It is not claimed that all who seek spirit healing are wholly cured instantly. It is claimed that the number of healings now numbers millions. The totals and percentages will be given in their proper place. That there are other aspects of healing there is no doubt. They speak for themselves. That there are variables, due mainly to the variable gifts of healers, there is no doubt; that is where the art of the healers in the realm beyond comes into play. If all healers were as effective as the best the total of hospitals would be much reduced and much money diverted to other purposes pressing on mankind.

Healing is not only a remedy for disease conditions. It penetrates the whole consciousness of man since its effects begin to show in the spirit of the individual seeking relief. In that way spirit healing is a reforming and spiritualising force. We work for improved, more humane, more kindly societies in which all kinds of poverty may be diminished so that the spirit will express itself more fully. These are considerations to be developed.

We claim that spirit healing also teaches that we need not live in crises and emergencies. It teaches that we may live more fully and fruitfully than ever before. We look for relief from many social problems, and in all, move towards a spiritualised world based upon demonstrated spiritual truths beginning with Survival and now emerging as healing for the whole human race, when it chooses to walk that path.

What has been happening in the scientific world? Has it made progress towards a healing concept such as outlined above? No. Science is persuaded, but not as firmly as before, that it must proceed by the way it has come: materialistic, experimental, seeking knowledge of nature's physical laws and forces and applying, through technology, the products of knowledge. No wise person would dream of questioning the achievements of science; for good and ill, since we should not forget that the science of war and killing marches with the science of health and education.

If science had satisfied the needs of mankind in the healing arts alone there would not have been such amendments as chiropractic, osteopathic, herbal, homeopathic, Christian Science and the rest of the scroll of remedies for what ails us. Some of the new ideas are truly revivals of ancient ideas. Even ancient China has opened some minds with acupuncture. Modern medical research missed that one.

It is a question: whether the discovery of one idea may prevent discovery of another equally effective idea once put to the test. The mesmerists were, no doubt, magnetic healers while some of them, equally without doubt, were spiritual healers who did not know the origin of their gifts. A place has been given to the hypnotists who are, at last, admitted to have a function in some aspects of healing. But there is no question that spirit healing is established; science cannot long ignore that truth. In its acquisitive zeal the medical profession has adopted therapies it could not legislate out of existence.

All of the foregoing leads to the conviction that the modern healing mission was planned by and is being carried out by our fellows in the spirit world in cooperation with us. All the evidence points to that view. I believe the drive was intended, first, to establish Survival. Once that concept was rooted strongly in human thought, the next phase was to increase the mission of the healers. That, in my lifetime alone, is demonstrated.

Now, the aim of the healing mission is not only to heal the sick of all disease manifestations but to develop thought to the point where these truths cannot ever again be dislodged. There have been many attempts in history to do what is now being done so well—and they were defeated almost wholly by the resistance exerted by those who profit most in power when they control the minds of the human race. We are beyond the initial stages. Comes now the task of showing that the wonderful physical body through which we express ourselves is what the poet Alexander Pope sang: the greatest study of mankind is man. He means by that the questions of God and the universe are beyond us, therefore, we should look inward. This has been done to a degree in all ages; now it is for all citizens of the world to benefit from newer aspects of the truth of both our bodies and our holy trinity: the spirit (or soul), the psychic nature and the physical body.

It is not necessary for my purpose to compress a view of the history of medicine into a few pages to make the next point. First, a short preliminary statement, then two examples of current developments which should shed some light on this vast subject.

When, later, you read my views on the consciousness of cells in the human body, the drift of the argument may not have been as clear as intended. I refer to the claim that every unit in the body is organised beyond human understanding and has its own distinct consciousness. This must be so else we could not function as we do now with all our aches, pains and disorders. Even in disease there is organisation, and intelligence and direction—or there could not be healing.

We cannot consciously direct a single cell in its functions. And there are billions upon billions of cells always at work, without pause on the tasks designed for and assigned to them. I am aware of the feats of some men, and women, who have devoted lifetimes to being able by mental discipline and directed will to raise or lower blood pressure, to raise and lower body temperature. This is not the same as directing the still largely incomprehensible cells at their multitude of tasks. The cellular and other activities are carried on whatever our physical positions, whether we are asleep or awake, whether we walk or run, stand up or sit down, are calm or agitated, are relaxed or tense, angry or benign, eating or fasting, thinking or feeling, taking in nourishment or excreting wastes, circulating blood or any other required liquid.

Where is the computer concept to carry such programmes as will keep us functioning? We have not yet considered the marvellous brain. Then there is the debated mind. Whence comes its power? Is it physical, psychic and/or spiritual?

Man is a universe contained within a body that may be graceful as a swan if we dance, inert as a fallen tree as we sleep. And all depends upon the harmonious life within a skin that is a wonder of wonders in its self-healing functions and responses to touch. What of the eye? The movement of a single finger? We cannot pause to talk of the wonder of a smile, or a caressing word. All of this and no consciousness, no design, no superior director—the person subject to his instrument, his body? All, all flesh and only conditioned flesh and no spirit?

Omitted from this treatment are the chemical factories within the body, the nervous systems, the grace of the body's movements, the marvels of the senses. Throughout all, the cellular complex is at work, coming to birth (how?), serving designed functions, responding with inexplicable speed and accuracy to all demands, dying, being renewed (how?), all to achieve and, if we permit it, by wise living, achieving the harmony called health. And all of this is within the empire and consciousness of a single person. The mind will take us farther. Indeed, we have some advanced scientific testimony tending to the view that the brain alone is superior to our new-found computer art.

When we have done with that, how do we determine where memory lives and how we may recall some of the stored information sometimes with flashing ease and at others wait for days for an answer? The questions are unending; the answers slow to come.

More and more we see references to the individuality of cells. This is a logical growth out of our increasing knowledge. We reason that anything so complex, so small, so essential has to be special since it is beyond our power to understand it now, and then only in part. The more we work at it the more we learn of the cells and the more we ask, why and how? How is much easier than why.

There are recent reports of specialists in cancer research speculating on the individuality of cells. Elsewhere others talk of teaching cancer patients to "think" their way to betterment at least by adopting the view that cells may be influenced by thought. To admit validity is the first step towards the probable, despite the catch-all view of a god of random chance.

It must be that increased awareness of spirit healing is

affecting scientific, and especially, medical thought since there are problems that do not respond to orthodox approaches, neither are such diseases as cancer yielding to current therapies as they should considering the vast research programmes over many years. The figures tell their own story. More people are dying of cancer.

The concept will one day be adopted in general thought that life is consciousness and consciousness is life, that everything is alive, filled with creative energy if we but knew how to release and employ it as it is utilised in every act of spirit healing.

Once establish the idea of the individuality of the cell, as a basis, and the power of materialism over thought will have to yield to wider, deeper, wiser concepts. The changes following then will be greater than even those arising from scientific effort over the centuries. It would be a first step across the physical boundary into the state of the metaphysical, or psychic.

Many wonder about the apparent adaptability of cells in the course of developing disease; adapting to medical efforts at control; developing "new" forms of disease; changes in environment by way of improvements in sanitation, diet, cleanliness and the like yet the total of sufferers from disease in general does not decrease. We have the medical preventive arts, the equipment to keep many alive who otherwise would be dead and demands for more hospitals and research increase.

Disease has become such a problem that governments of most societies find they must subsidise medical care otherwise the health of millions would deteriorate still further. When public medicine is adopted by societies where not many years ago it was an act of disloyalty to a political creed, then we have an admission that disease is a major industry. It is a comment on societies as a whole that they seldom act save from immediate need or in the face of a crisis which could have been prevented.

That method of treatment which will reduce sickness among humans as individuals, and as societies will, in time, command citizen loyalty. The preventive measures do not appear to work well, as in the case of cancer, the world's "fear" disease, so there must be something basically wrong with the way we live and the way we force the physical system to "adapt", one adaptation being cancer. A paradox: we learn most about health when we are diseased.

Yet a non-medical pioneer, Harry Edwards, has long since been persuaded, based upon some 15 million healings, mostly at a distance, that cells are individuals, that they have consciousness, that they respond perfectly to our states of nutrition, hygiene, love, hate, fear, frustration; they are what we think and feel because they are of the matrix of our bodies and our psychic natures and of our physical natures and our spiritual natures. The holy trinity is everywhere until the day we shed the physical body. When we disturb the harmony of our threefold being, the disease follows, whether by any fear or irremediable frustration.

It is strange that the boundary between the physical and the metaphysical, or in this instance, the psychic, has been crossed so often by multitudes that most of the great intellects of our ages have either not perceived the fact or have avoided considering it. You would think that intellectuals do so much thinking that they would have found a way to inquire into the reality of other states of consciousness, apart from drugs. The phenomena are there, always there. That's where it all begins for we citizens of this planet.

There is no measure of the loss accrued by humanity through the refusal of scientists to look into our claims, although privately many have benefited from our demonstrations of healing and of Survival. Perhaps scientists are not more advanced than we are; perhaps their distinction is that they specialise in specific areas about which we know little, therefore, we regard them with some awe—until we look at their overall impact on mankind. It is a comfort, almost, restores a balance of values, when you ponder that though a respected scientist, or even a bishop or a pope, may not in a lifetime be aware of the world beyond this one, yet many humble, unnamed citizens are regular visitants there.

The Lord of Life moves in mysterious ways his wonders to perform.

You may recall that Benjamin Franklin, who was not accepted as a scientist, was an enterprising experimenter in physical phenomena. When he flew a kite, with a heavy metal key attached, a doubting woman asked him what was the use of it. He replied with: "What use is a new born baby?" The baby was an experiment in conducting lightning to ground. It was a baby thought and much came of it. So are the thoughts of cells as conscious entities with individualities.

Without being expert in any medical or scientific field, we may discuss some scientific and medical situations. Among them is one concerning not the cellular but the consciousness question. It also has much to do with the nature of matter which used to be the rock of materialist theory. To discuss such questions we, again, have to digress for a little venture into a difficult field: psychics and physicists, or psychics and the famous scientists. I have been there before. A return visit showed how much progress has been made in the consciousness affair.

(A personal reflection: since becoming aware that my speculations on consciousness were anticipated by a colleague whom I respect and admire, I feel more kindly towards cells and so on. I have to confess I feel better now that I realise just how important it is that my billions of internal friends are working for my benefit.

A little reciprocity does not hurt. Think well of them.)

Just as in the healing story I felt the need to trace growth from biblical times forward to obtain perspective and to look once more at the signposts, so I looked back to the golden age of scientific research into psychic phenomena produced through the gifts of celebrated mediums of the Victorian times. These mediums beat a path for the healers.

At the height of the materialist age, from the beginning of the 19th century to the first half of the 20th century, eminent scientists, literary figures and statesmen were involved in psychic research at a level not matched since that time. In a later period the impact of the psychic interest reached even the theologians. Scientists were involved in disputes, some of them equal in eminence in their own fields to those of the small group which made psychic history. Controversy over the universal question of Survival became heated to the point that it aroused opinion all over Britain, spread to the United States, and to the most advanced nations in Europe.

Queen Victoria always had a medium with her. Her personal servant, a highlander, John Brown, was, much later, alleged to have been her lover. Instead he was a medium with whom she held meetings so that her beloved Prince Albert could talk with her. Imagine: the British Empire being run from the spirit world! Brown had been recommended to the queen by another famous medium, R. J. Lees, who, among things, was responsible for the arrest of the insane surgeon responsible for the Jack the Ripper murders. The documents in that case are still impounded. The killer's name is still withheld. When Queen Victoria died the Bishop of Winchester, Dr. Randall Davidson, burned some of the queen's diaries in which she, it is claimed, had recorded her seances with John Brown.

In the same general period President Lincoln always had a medium in the White House. It is stated in a book written by one of his mediums that during the Civil War it was under spirit guidance that the great president acted to issue his proclamation freeing the slaves. That book, *Was Abraham a Spiritualist?*, says the American spirits who counselled Lincoln urged his signing the proclamation as commander-in-chief and forecast that if he did so, victory would follow. He did so. Victory followed.

In the scientific field the already famous scientist, Sir William Crookes, undertook a study of materialisation phenomena as produced through the mediumship of Florence Cook. Crookes, who was in the course of his career twice President of the British Association for the Advancement of Science, was hailed by the London *Times* in an editorial which said that now the British people would get the truth, or falsity, of the claims of Spiritualists. Crookes found, in many experiments carried out in the orthodox scientific manner, that the claims were true, and he so proved it. He had himself photographed arm in arm with a materialised young woman, Katie King, and tested the effect of a force emanating from the medium which activated scientific testing equipment. Crookes was a noted experimenter, an innovative chemist, physicist and for his labour in that field, presumably, was knighted by Queen Victoria. Sir Arthur Conan Doyle, creator of Sherlock Holmes, a Spiritualist leader, was honoured at the same time. Their first meeting was when Queen Victoria honoured them.

The student is referred to my little book on the subject, *Science in the Seance Room*, long out of print. Its merit is as a compilation of the successes of some scientists and of classic experiments in psychic phenomena.

Then there are the contributions of Sir Alfred Russel Wallace, a man born in humble circumstances who, by his vision and endurance, made a contribution to science which may be ranked with Newton's although in a vastly different field. Newton sought the harmony of nature in the world of gigantic forces and discovered their majestic laws; Wallace, and with him Darwin, sought nature's laws in the development of species. Darwin was the private man in his writing; Wallace, more physically adventurous, was a public man.

Wallace worked alone, for years, in the perilous jungles and forests of Malaya for explanations of the origin of the species. He is the independent discoverer of the process of natural selection. Public praise in the mid-19th century went to Darwin; Wallace was scarcely mentioned. He went to the wrong school. His discovery came as he lay in a fever on an island off New Guinea, weakened by years of privation. In his search for an explanation of the origin of species, he had a flashing insight. He had been pondering the massive destruction in nature, the casualties among mankind by disease, war, accident or famine. Then, in his own words: "Vaguely thinking over the enormous and constant destruction this implied, it occurred to me to ask the question, 'Why do some die and some live?'." He produced the answer: "The best fitted to live: From the effects of disease the most healthy escaped; from the enemies the strongest, the swiftest, or the most cunning; from the famine, the best hunters."

He followed this by the view that all the required changes needed for adaptation of the species would be developed over long periods and the changes would be made as the environment changed . . . the fittest to survive would emerge in every generation.

Darwin had written the same views in England, 10,000 miles away. He had not published them. In June, 1858, Darwin received Wallace's excited letter from distant Malaysia telling of his discovery. Darwin had stated his discovery in almost identical terms in a private letter to a colleague some years earlier. There was no conflict over priority, a marked change from the behaviour today of some in the scientific world where the conduct and grab for fame resembles the scrambles of the market place. Darwin was magnanimous in his praise of Wallace's superior presentation of the new theory. The subsequent upheaval in scientific thought brought by these two giants has not yet been exhausted.

That is one more signpost in the development of the thought of the world.

Revelation comes by progressive discovery based upon unremitting work and penetrating mental effort. At that point the muse of inspiration acts—and the new idea is born only to be changed and illuminated later by other explorers. Great discoveries close eras of thought; they do not inaugurate eras. The thought completed, the way opens up for the revelation following. So the continuing process works its will and mankind is changed because its thought is changed. The body holds to its nature in the flesh but is the more receptive of its invisible components.

Before Wallace left his worldwide laboratory he had grown intellectually, I believe largely because of his psychic and spiritual experiences. He was in his early days a powerful mesmerist, witnessed demonstrations of surgery done under hypnosis and knew well how the human functions and qualities respond to what is properly called human magnetism.

I believe it was his powerfully developed psychic nature that led him naturally, but with scientific training, to his discoveries. I believe his psychic nature taught him to be open-minded in an age coming into its first, profound changes. He stepped forward from materialism into the realm of thought and of change and of insight into the workings of nature.

Before he left this earth Wallace moved towards an enlarged view of the origin of species; he speculated that a telepathic process aided the development. Few contemporary biologists now incline to that view.

He was unafraid of controversy. In a forthright statement during the continuing dispute over his psychic convictions he wrote: "The whole history of science shows us that, whenever the educated and scientific men of any age have denied the facts of other investigators on *a priori* grounds of absurdity or impossibility, the pioneers have always been right."

He was right on both grounds, psychic and scientific.

Many of us now in what are called the golden years have witnessed demonstrations of psychic phenomena at the visual and "solid" level and we cannot erase the impact made on our thinking. I recall, as a part of a lifetime apprenticeship, being in a group with Harry Edwards, the famous healer, when his close friend, Jack Webber, a remarkable physical medium, was the instrument for a demonstration.

Webber was tightly roped into a heavy chair, his jacket was stiched so that he could not take it off. He was entranced and levitated to the ceiling of the large room in which we met. We saw Webber elevated above the heads of the audience. Meanwhile his spirit guide made comments in a voice distinct from the medium's when in his normal state. When Webber was returned to his chair, his jacket was as we had left it, the stitches intact, the ropes in position—yet Webber had left that chair, his jacket was removed—yet, he, and the jacket, were as we left them when examined as the seance ended.

An explanation of the processes involved, from the material point of view, is too involved to detail here; yet it was a clear experiment defying the known laws of materialist physics. In addition, there are further complex questions as to what happened to Webber during such a demonstration. These questions must bear on the subject before us: the nature and powers of the psychic world. Miracles are no explanation; miracles are excuses for lack of reason and evidence.

The phenomena just described in its many manifestations is of a piece with healing; they emanate from the same source and bear clear evidence of superior and still unexplained control over both mind and matter. On reflection it seems that Edwards' development as a healer and his understanding of psychic phenomena was aided through his association with Webber and other physical mediums.

Then there was the outstanding mediumship of Helen Duncan, victim of a clumsy prosecution under the ancient and since repealed Witchcraft Act on a charge of "conjuration of spirits". And that in a society which does not formally accept the existence of spirits although their claimed reality is the basis of the Christian and all other religions. The court found Duncan guilty on the ground of fraud, thereby leading to a successful campaign by Spiritualists for repeal of the act and the enactment of another—the Fraudulent Mediums Act. As the only journalist who reported the case from its first stage to the appeal court I believe there could have been a better defence. Yet, in the atmosphere of ignorance of the phenomena, prejudice had to win. I also believe that Helen Duncan's death was hastened by her being imprisoned. A close friend who visited her in jail agrees with that view.

It now appears that the Duncan case signalled another stage in the long evolution of the spirit mission. The publicity within a nation then fighting for its life was almost incredible. But it marked a turning point. From then on healing became the centre of interest. Few materialisation mediums are available for demonstrations now. I believe the change was designed. The road to a surge in healing was opened as the jail doors closed on Helen Duncan, a great pioneer in the greatest of all causes.

What is the position of the scientist in all of the foregoing? The words of Sir Alfred Russel Wallace sound again: "The pioneer when he has the facts is always right". We have the facts. Scientists are reluctant even to examine them, save on their own terms. Even when that is agreed there are always the after-thoughts and the expected relapse or remissions into complacency. Yet, we must not confuse science with scientists.

We have so little physical power in this world, we who follow our convictions of the existence of another life. Those who serve the expectations of the market place and the policies of governments include scientists since without their efforts there could not be any wars. Their defence is clear: they serve. Our case is clear also: we serve without killing. Our mission is to heal the body and the mind. The day will come when science no longer serves as a weapon for war but for peace and for the removal of poverty and disease everywhere.

If we could but enlist the steady attention of scientists to examine our experience and our case the world would greatly benefit. You have seen how a few bold, pioneering scientists in another era changed thought over a wide area in the psychic and physical world. There can be no going back. Their discoveries are but the groundwork for others yet to come.

Some of the most eminent men and women in science are compelled to admit that the frontier of matter has been reached. This obliges the most adventurous thinkers who are unafraid to speak their thoughts on such a sweeping change. Men of the standing of Jeans and Eddington, of recent fame, and Planck of contemporary fame, say there is no opening seen so far beyond matter unless they turn, as Planck writes, to the metaphysical. He does not mean that in a mystical sense but as a further state beyond matter. Other thinkers say we are left with thought only, when all is considered; I take that to mean in the face of the discoveries in atom physics. I would like to be able to say that they had seen the light and had come to understand the nature of some psychic laws. They will see that light some day—perhaps through understanding of the laws and energies upon which healing is developed.

There is accumulating evidence of certain aspects of spirit healing which may open some scientific eyes, whether by increasing results, wider practice of healing, or a development in techniques of measuring the effects of such healing. To make such a prophecy is not to take on the mantle of the penetrating seer; the probability that this is the path that will be followed is implicit in all previous advances in healing; revelation is as progressive as formal theorising, followed by experiment. There is more than one way to acquire knowledge.

Allegiance to matter as being all there is, must weaken as more knowledge becomes available, and comes through studies of the healers at work. It would be desirable if we could find a small group of, say, younger scientists with an awareness of some psychic promptings, to take the plunge and by developing as healers apply their analytic skills—as knowers and doers. In this way, but not the only way, the bridge between matter and the metaphysical may be crossed as scientists are already accustomed to crossing bridges between the known and the about-to-be-known.

I say, as you would expect, that we and multitudes of others have crossed that bridge in personal experiences or have clear knowledge through psychic phenomena and through changes in our own consciousness. One day we will be in the majority of those who know. That weight of opinion will do much to change thought—which according to the scientific trend is all we have.

Even the achievements of scientists in space research do not touch the human questions. They have not dealt with supersitition—and fear. Orthodoxy is a hard nut to crack before we can get at the meat of it. Yet, the plain man may be dimly aware of a metaphysical world without being able to articulate what he dimly perceives. There is a reason. The mind cannot cause us to know or even dimly perceive what is beyond our capacity to receive. How is the mind to impress the brain save by impulses, if not from within the mind, then by experiences outside the mind? For example: we who are not art conscious nor music conscious may learn, stage by stage, to begin to appreciate art. Similarly we may come to like music, in any form, even the crudest, as a matter of choice—once we are immersed in artistic or musical activities.

That is the process: bombardment of the consciousness by concepts until a pathway is made in the mind, that wonder of wonders with its subordinate, the brain, executing the marvellous adaptability displayed even by the seemingly simple act of breathing. It is thus that the bridge between the physical and the spiritual is built out of the psychic nature. Across that bridge the communication flows both ways, day and night, always functioning as we give it means to persist; responding to every stimulus and with a magic we only now begin to appraise, giving us our humanity and preserving us on our journey across this life.

That bridge, the psychic bridge, was already formed when the first man as we know him walked this earth. His psychic nature had to be developed before he took flesh for a garment of experience else he could not maintain his link with his mind, his ruler, governor and guide. In the ensuing aeons man lost intimate contact with his psychic nature though it maintained and now increasingly maintains its compact as a member of the trinity of the physical, the psychic and the spiritual. This has always been man's position through all of his physical evolution.

Man has always been crossing the frontier between the two worlds because that is his nature. He is not always, nor even often, aware of the secret he carries with him in every breath he draws, every step he takes, every thought he utters, every emotion he feels, every condition of love or hate he experiences. Where physical science pauses intellectually on the brink, pondering whether to make the leap from the physical into the oceans of the metaphysical, the plain man—and the scientist—are experiencing the metaphysical every moment, only the awareness is low-ebbed because of overlays of erroneous views called orthodoxy. We, all of us, have to bear the burdens of our civilisation. We are shaped by all manner of environments. These have to be taken into account when we assess ourselves in relation to any discovery of our inward natures.

There come times when we doubt what we are beginning to know. We thereby delay our understanding. But use and custom of learning to listen to our own minds and psychic intimations will, in due time, bring us to the realisation that we are what is here declared—spirits now and forever, indestructible, but for a time and for an experience to grow, wearing a wonderful robe of flesh.

It is into that world that science must one day go. To continue round upon round of experiment upon experiment on the nature of matter will not, of itself, bring us to the doors of the dwelling of the spirit. Once we are aware of these inward things we begin our great adventure. That road is hardest of all since it cannot be made smooth by the flesh, nor by distressing the body nor making coarse the emotions. By living towards the best we know we slowly mature, ready to take the first step on the homeward road.

By its neglect of the physical phenomena proving the existence of a psychic world science has lost great opportunities. Much would have been learned about the mind if science had not fused it with its physical organ, the brain, and that fusion again with what scientists vaguely call the spirit, a kind of nimbus kept in an intellectual limbo to be brought out at some unspecified time for examination.

Confusion over the brain/mind will begin to be cleared up when the identity of these distinct but co-operative organs are understood. It is easy to challenge and scoff at the views of those outside the science field and say they do not know there is a separate mind. Perhaps we do not but, at least, we have facts amounting to persuasive evidence. I call it proof for reasons already stated—articulate, intelligent speech from a materialised entity showing all the faculties of we solid humans. If the speech is as described then it cannot proceed from the medium asleep in trance. The evidence is there: science will not look at it, and there is nothing we can do about it until science comes out of its materialistic trance that there is but one world, the fleshy, the material, the measurable, the tangible, the moving, breathing, speaking, singing, dancing, communicating wonder called man. He is not the end of evolution. He can be and is simulated in psychic materialisation, proving the brain is not the mind, unless a brain is also duplicated, wonder enough to cause alarm in the academies of scientific learning.

There are many books on the brain/mind. Neurologists tell us much about the brain's operation, the marvels of the neural systems. That is not challenged. They have yet to show us there is no intelligence apart from the brain, even without its hyphenated twin, the mind. We should here recall the statement by Sir Alfred Russel Wallace about the rigidity of science and the value of the pioneer with facts in advance of orthodox teaching.

Once it is clearly established that the mind is a distinct organ superior to the brain since it survives death we are again in the non-physical realm of consciousness. The mind and brain are not opponents; they are units of a whole, the mind being the superior because that is its function—to express the soul. The mind is superior because it is closer to the realm of causes, or, if you prefer it that way, closer to the source of creativity. This concept is not difficult to ponder; all that is required is evidence. This abounds in the areas already covered.

This exposition, with its evangelism, is not far removed from the current frontier attitude of the eminent in science. Since this is planned as a layman's view, I shall not try to write in technical terms. All outstanding scientists write clearly since their aim in their work is to see clearly. I do not propose to load this story with references, but the following will stand for many:

A recent Nobel Prize winner, Prof. Salvador E. Luria, Director of the Centre for Cancer Research, Massachusetts Institute of Technology, urged, in a recent literary magazine article, that scientists should continue research "comparable only to the successes of physics in the first quarter of this century" (a reference probably to the advances in atomic physics). He says that successes of the kind he had in mind have begun to find ". . . direct application to cancer and other diseases". That is welcome news. How much success is being achieved is not stated in the incomplete report I have. Luria writes of the brain after stating that a biology of the mind "is feasible and is one of the great goals of science, possibly the greatest".

Could so eminent a scientist be confusing mind with

brain? Of the brain he says, contrary to what others have said, "... it is not a computer, grows, is made new in each individual, starting from the instructions from the genes, which provide a specific chemical programme for the brain as for any other organ . . . the brain's creativity is beyond the combinational possibilities of any computer if nothing else because of the thousands of billions of nerve cells in the brain."

Somewhere farther back it was asserted that the child is born with its own matrix upon which it develops: the foundation on which the life of the individual is built. Is that so different from Luria's view? If he can push back the line separating his programme from a matrix, not physical but psychic, we may be thinking about the same situation. The scientist generally is wedded to cells, which in itself is a revolution so absorbing that many outstanding scientists may be lost in wonder at their complexity.

In part, this is Luria's conclusion: "... I believe a real relevance of science is to cultivate . . . a vision of the resolution of the great mysteries of nature . . . we gain if we connect our work with some further, grander goal..."

Could the grander goal have been reached without science being aware of it? Could Russel Wallace be smiling?

That so distinguished a scientist as Luria should identify mind with brain is disconcerting since he also talks of the wonder of the brain's "creativity". Does he mean that creativity arises from brain cells and nerves alone, even thousands of billions of them?

Luria's statements seem to be paving the way for a distant method of isolating the brain to discover the source and system of brain creativity, just as other researchers claimed to have found that memory is retained in brain tissue? That claim was withdrawn.

The Nobel Prize winner speaks of "coming to grips with the most intriguing feature of the creativity of the human spirit." Thus we have a choice of three organs—the mind, the brain and the spirit. This is not to infer that he is coming over to our side, only that, for all his eminence, he is in some difficulty with his terms since there is no place in scientific classifications for what he says about spirit, mind and creativity.

His views take another turn: ". . . one needs to understand the 'individuality' of nerve cells that causes a given fibre, from the eye for example, to make a precise connection with a cell or group of cells in the lower brain, which, in turn, send their fibres precisely to certain columns of brain cells in the brain cortex."

Without seeming to don the mantle of a neurologist I take that to mean what Edwards says, that cells, like all other wonders of the human body, have their individuality and distinct states of consciousness, billions of them. Edwards' conviction stems from 45 years of spirit healing; education by the spirit does the rest. Edwards is convinced that cells are individualities and that the discord we set up in them—the unresolved frustrations, tensions, and fears trigger the chain reactions which we call disease.

I have a description by a medical researcher of the selectivity of cells. He cites, as an example, a portion of an upper arm, damaged and of the healing process that ensues. The cells in command of the affected area wait by the cellular stream, looking for desired cells to repair what was lost. These waiting cells use what may be a hook-like part to seize the desired cells, probably in their millions, as they race past and incorporate them into the healing process. No other kind of cell is taken. This, if it is a true report of some process observed (and I do not see what is to be gained by misreporting), indicates selectivity which indicates intelligence. Since this occurs in one area observed, why not elsewhere?

It is not essential that we are aware every second of the

day of all the processes in our bodies. We do not have the capability, therefore, what is called the creative intelligence sets up automatic systems, programmed to carry out specific functions. If we co-operate by providing suitable conditions, in all respects, the body will be well; if we break the pattern the system's sensors respond to trigger corrective action. Then we have the conditions we call disease. To anyone professional in the area this is not a far-out statement. They might agree, except that they would invoke a random chance explanation of a first cause. That way no progress lies for it is hard to see how disorder can produce the magnificent order that makes our bodies so inexplicably designed.

Now that a Nobel Prize winner, Prof. Luria, urges research into the biology of the brain/mind, there comes to attention a long report of experiments by medical researchers into healing given by a retired Hungarian army colonel, who is called Mr. E. but is Oskar Estebany. The report makes the usual genuflections in the direction of charges of charlatanry in healing (usually associated with psychic matters but not with scientific research into psychic matters); there is a difference, as will be seen. But, you are assured that in the following summary the scientists write about just plain healing without the word "psychic" to show that all is as it should be. Only, like all else in the universe, everything God makes, or creates, has a crack in it. So has the report on Mr. E's healing gift.

Mr. E has a way with animals. When he rode in the Hungarian army he found that sick horses recovered faster with him than with others.

Mr. E has been news for many years with his healing merely by laying on hands. He is not deeply devout, as the newspapers say, with their instruments for measuring devotion, nor does he pray before healing. The healings occur. He does not, he says, appeal to God.

The story begins with a lecture by Dr. Bernard Grad, a biochemist of McGill University, Montreal, Canada. He told of Mr. E just laying hands on wounded mice (that is, mice wounded in a laboratory by experimenters) and on distressed barley seeds. The results astonished the mice, no doubt, they also astonished Dr. Justa Smith, a nun and nutritionist specialising in enzymes, the substance which changes all metabolic reactions within cells without itself being changed (a catalyst).

Dr. Grad's lecture was delivered in 1966. The news of Mr. E's successful healing seems to have been delayed on the road to becoming communication.

Anyway, some wounded mice were treated by Mr. E and by some non-healers who just went through their role laying of on hands and some were treated by nothing at all; just the motions. Mr. E's treated mice "healed significantly faster" than two other groups in the experiment. He also produced significant growth in distressed seeds.

Dr. Smith was urged by Dr. Grad to test the healer with enzymes because of her skill in that area. She had already "dumbfounded" (that's what the report says) her colleagues by showing that magnetic fields applied to an enzyme solution had shown substantially increased activity. The next step: Mr. E was wired to a special thermometer to maintain temperature at a constant level to determine whether heat alone would affect the enzyme solution. A report of that experiment shows:

An enzyme solution was exposed to ultraviolet light at a highly damaging wavelength long enough to reduce activity by about 25 percent to test the healer's ability to restore its activity. He did so, as to 90 percent in half an hour. Dr. Smith said he could have restored the enzyme to 100 percent.

In tests to increase the effect of a magnetic field, Mr. E

raised it to a point at least 16,000 times more than that of the earth. No magnetic field was found to be emanated from his hands.

So much for the carefully instrumented and monitored tests of the effects of Mr. E's power, whatever scientists may theorise it to be. There was, to me, a much more significant test. The chief of staff of a Buffalo, N.Y., hospital asked Dr. Smith to take Mr. E to the bedside of a woman said by him to be "clinically at the point of death". After only two treatments by Mr. E the woman was released from the hospital. Dr. Justa Smith is also a nun. If this heightens the value of her testimony, it is in the report.

Leaving aside the effect of Mr. E's successes with seeds, mice and magnetic fields, it is clear that his success with the woman said to be "clinically at the point of death" is the more important—and striking as well as the most illuminating. But the emphasis of all discussions of his work is on the seeds, the poor wounded mice, and the magnetic fields. You might have thought the healing of the dying woman was the more important—without instrumentation.

To summarise: Dr. Smith, a venturesome scientist, looked at healing objectively and says: "It is possible that the energy Mr. E exerts may eventually be found somewhere in the electromagnetic spectrum". It is more likely, she says, it is an energy still unnamed. She speculates that it may be a life force and adds that only a tiny portion of the macro-molecule of an enzyme is required for its catalytic function.

If, as she speculates, the energy used in healing is either in the electro-magnetic spectrum or is an unnamed energy, why has the massive research by physicists not found what appears a regular phenomenon with Mr. E? Lack of interest by scientists is easy to anticipate. It is remarkable that Dr. Grad and Dr. Smith were so open-minded. The speculations of Dr. Smith are the more progressive.

I go farther; it is inevitable that science will discover that the secret is in the direction of the human healer being the catalyst and the transmitter of psychic energy; that the human being will be hailed at some not far distant time as the wonderful agent for the transmission of healing. There, I am persuaded, is the place to look, even if it means liberating mice from their unsought sacrifice in the interests of science.

I have often wondered in studies in healing how the wonderfully delicate nerves, when severed in surgery, "know" how to reconnect themselves. In my sole experience as a privileged spectator at eye surgery I reasoned that the nerves must be instructed, or knew what to do, since there was no sign that the surgeons did anything that would show how the reconnecting was done. I asked the senior surgeon, a friend, who had at one time sought healing for himself, how he explained it. He said it was one of nature's mysteries. And we left it at that—then.

I have since reasoned, reinforced by Edwards' teaching, derived from his experience and instructons from healers, doctors and scientists in the spirit that the universe is consciousness, that intelligence—and knowledge—is everywhere, just as energy is everywhere. Both consciousness and energy will be better understood one day and mankind will then have some better answers to its two questions: how and why. It is by persistent searching that we will come to know more of the fuller life and on the way we will learn to live in harmony, all people, all nations, all nature and all spirit. It will be worth working for through the ages now forming in the mists of the becoming.

This leads directly from the statement by Prof. Luria and the much earlier conviction reached by Edwards, gathered during his long career as healer-scientist. On a lesser scale I had arrived at such a view although some 21 years absent from England and not directly involved in healing. In our few letters I had sought healing for others, at their request, from Edwards, yet our positions regarding consciousness as prevalent everywhere and directed by intelligence everywhere coincided. Edwards was in contact with tens of thousands of people; I live a quiet life in a quiet place, seeing only a few persons, with occasional excursions into the hustle and bustle. How, then, did Edwards and I come to like opinions? Not by direct personal contact, I believe, but by being in contact, mentally with spirit teachers of the same persuasion who impressed ideas as we moved towards them in our seeking? The bald explanation of telepathy, or the direct transfer of thought from mind to mind is not sufficient although it may be a beginning of an explanation. I hold that there is another and superior method, open to all: a kind of mental absorption from a spirit source of thought from which we may draw when our natures are attuned to it. It is, I believe, that from this ocean of thought we may receive ideas shaped by our spirit co-operators.

It is easy to see why materialistic physics having practically and philosophically reached a frontier, that the most penetrating minds should turn to one of two directions—an attempt to cross the frontier into the metaphysical on a basis not yet developed, or to turn to further studies in biology in the hope of finding answers there. It is no hazard to predict which will succeed now, or at all, but the probabilities, based upon experience, are that the scientific move will be towards the biological. That is closest to the wholly physical; the move towards the metaphysical involves other than scientists. In that way the scientist loses control, forgetting that he cannot control the planets yet makes discoveries about them.

In the tendency towards a new biology, there will be emphasis on the nature of the brain/mind, since the mental atmosphere has been somewhat cleared of materialist prejudice against the validity of anything psychic, unless you count the elementary and near-physical experiments in what is called extra-sensory perception.

Once the biologists, or others, have developed extended views of the brain/mind they are confronted with the validity of the concept of "individuality" of cells. If "individuality" is valid for cells, why not for enzymes and the other components or appearances of the body's constituents? Materialist science is at a crossroads. It may oscillate between positions; if it is to cross the boundary to the metaphysical it will have to contend with the social consequences arising from even a minor success. Once over the frontier there is no force in the universe that could halt the consequent revolution that must burst upon the world: that what has been a phrase, the mind, is become a reality, that the unseen is now seen, in its phenomena if not in pictures, but seen by its effects which must change all other concepts.

Whether we who now consider these matters will be on earth to witness the revolution of thought is doubtful. In another environment we will see, with some satisfaction, I hope, that another giant step has been taken in the progress of mankind towards liberation from the earth as the sole condition of life.

SCIENCE SEARCHES FOR "UNSEEN FORCE" AS AN EXPLANATION OF HEALING

SPIRIT HEALERS ARE CATALYSTS FOR THE HEALING ENERGIES

## POSTSCRIPT TO SCIENCE SECTION

Now that two of the principal aspects of the healing art, and the philosophy derived from it, are stated, a summation is in order. You will recall that in the case of Mr. E, selected from among many and mainly for his topicality, the tests described were under controls established and supplied by the scientist named. The results stated by the scientist were so obviously impressive that she speculated not whether the phenomena were genuine—she could not honestly believe otherwise—but, what is the energy upon which the phenomena are founded?

That position of proof of psychic forces has been standard and developing for more than 130 years. Official science has not changed its neutral position despite the declarations by some of its most eminent men that the frontier of matter has been reached. In the Mr. E case the experimenter theorises that the energy upon which the phenomena are based "has not yet been named". Naming and understanding are not the same thing. But, once identification and utilisation are known—there we have a revolutionary discovery beyond those of Newton, Wallace and Einstein. Perhaps that is why the search for the unknown force takes so long. It probably is so because mentally we are not yet at the stage of awareness required to grasp, understand and apply such a force. Since man's record of misuse of natural and human resources is by Cain's hand stamped invisibly on every brow, we may have far to go before we are beyond the darkness we have fashioned by our misdeeds. This is not to argue nicely a moral quantum factor, that is, little explosions of goodness, little but still good, emerging continuously but never sufficient to produce radical change.

The intellectual passion for classifying everything prevents even many leading experimenters in the physical sciences from advancing knowledge of the Spirit Science. Their basic error is that they treat the spirit as though it were an elusive form of matter. This is because they are of fixed minds, as the orthodox priest is fixed in his theology.

Spirit, not the vague Sunday-go-to-church thing, is real, more so than matter because matter is at the outer edge, the denser form assumed by spirit so that the processes of evolution are expressed. Matter cannot command Spirit for Spirit is the superior state. Therefore, the scientist cannot command the healer/medium. Scientists must, if they are to understand Spirit, come to the position of the healer/mediums.

Instead of persevering in the deep mines of matter, scientists must come up into the light of psychic and spiritual awareness. Then they will discover, through direct personal experience, what occurs when healing is at work. The truth of this knowledge cannot be known from the Outside; it is known only from the Inside of Consciousness.

Although there is much for healer/mediums to learn about the nature of the forces they receive and transmit, they are part of the process; they co-operate. The intellectual may scoff that this is asking for an act of faith through attunement. Whatever the description, the fact is always there. Intellect alone will not pry open the way to purely intellectual control of the processes of spirit healing.

The healing energy does not require to be classified

in order to be understood as a reality known by every healer/medium. That energy has its effects in healing in such manifestations that cannot be understood or explained by physical science.

Spirit healing is not an exercise in research at the outer limits of physics; it is a co-operative enterprise that involves the spiritual nature of man. It involves the mind and the heart, for at its root the nourishing substance is compassion.

Desired chemical changes in the physical body are achieved by spirit-directed thought into the patient's spirit mind, and through the brain beneficially by way of the physical mind.

Instead of seeking answers at the physical level in efforts to understand the phenomena of healing, scientists should encourage use of the power of imagination. The imagination is what the word says—the power to shape images of thought and emotion. In other times scientists sought to make models, mechanical models to express their ideas of the processes of nature and their world. More mature men among them changed that view until the modern views pushed their theorising to the limits of matter. And that, incontestably, is where they are today.

Scientists cannot make, or imagine Spirit, nor can they make a mechanical model of the healing processes because they are not at that level of consciousness where it can be known. Healer/mediums are aware of the changes in consciousness which signal the chemical changes in the body necessary to effect cures. The spirit energies involved have a counterpart in physical energies. As Planck, a great scientist, has stated, everything physical has a metaphysical counterpart. Change the word "metaphysical" to "spiritual", and our case is conceded. The role of the spirit energies is so to change their physical counterparts chemically that a healing is effected in the patient's body. In mental healing, the same process occurs.

Therefore, in brief, the awe in which physical science is now regarded by laymen should be transferred to the superior art and science of spiritual development. Healer/mediums cannot go to physical science; but physical science must raise its consciousness to a level of spirit awareness.

As electrical energy is reduced in power to a level where it may drive a motor, so spirit energy is transformed, by spirit beings, to that level at which, in turn, chemical changes occur in the human mind and body—and another healing is achieved.

Official science has no concept of the extent and range of healings achieved over the past decades alone. Spirit healing is changing human thought. In time it will be recognised as humanity's religion and the science and art of living.

The scientific "I will not know" position inhibits the mere prospect of knowing since scientists do not see prophetically what they seek with intellectual coldness—the discovery of an energy beyond their arts. What bedevils the scientific mind? They, the scientists, are the same in all recent centuries, in all cultures. They will not know unless the knowledge comes on their terms according to their rules.

There is little point in the scientist seeking from the healer/medium a scientific description of the energies transmitted through his consciousness since he does not know. But there are postulates which govern the science of spirit healing. These are set out in the Appendix. Is it a gland, or enzymes, or cells, or genes? Is it the psychic nature?

Scientists even now may be at work on theories of energies far beyond the crude, early release of energy in the first atomic bomb. We are by many deaths incurred far beyond that. Maybe scientists have a super-nuclear bear by the tail and cannot use it and cannot let go. It is unlikely that the healing energy is of such a destructive order since it is not within man's power to direct. It flows, as before said, but may not be commanded nor harnessed to men's wills. It cannot kill since it is benign and is in the safe keeping beyond the grasp of grasping men.

This, again, is a paradox: A healing force known by its benign effects, a healing corps, largely volunteer, trained (if that is the word) to become silent channels of a silent power that does not require even prayer, nor supplications, nor rituals, nor choirs, nor cathedrals but which flows at the call of need and pain and does not demand faith before nor loyalty afterwards.

The current situation has historic parallels, as witness the Biblical healings and healings in all cultures in all ages. A difference seen now is that science, having come to a stand on matter, is compelled to look beyond. Healer/mediums bridge the chasm between matter and spirit at each healing. In time it will be known how it is done, even as men now know of the genes, the enzymes, the cells and the nerves whereas before the body was a mystery and its chemistry unknown.

If in this situation we take refuge in the caves of superstition we could well be talking of mystery, miracle and magic. The wise, advanced souls in the spirit who have the healing mission in their care are resolved that since so many earlier missions were destroyed when men seized the instruments of reform that this will not happen again. How is such a situation to be achieved? By increasing not only the numbers of servers but to weave the knowledge of spirit truths into the very fabric of the mind of mankind, including the new science of the spirit in such close bond that they cannot again be dislodged. That is the position we have reached today, despite all the crudities and vulgarities displayed by the camp followers of the advancing armies of liberation.

Unless you have experienced the effects of the spirit

healing power it is not possible to credit fully the change of mind and emotion following. You may doubt many things later, you may even seek to persuade yourself you are mistaken but inwardly you know you are healed. You cannot undo what is done. The spirit healing is done. The evidence is insurmountable.

Only a historian of science could render a fair verdict upon the claim that science has never before shown such an obscuring face as the one she now wears. Is it due to fear that the heavens might fall if matter were deposed as ruler of the world's mind? Scientists should ponder their own case as humans.

We consciously control only the fewest and least of our functions, although by our actions, thoughts and emotions we deeply affect them. We are weak, physically, we are wayward (requiring continuous correction), we are born laboriously, we learn to walk upright slowly and with difficulty, we are slow in mental development, require a special environment to maintain our fragile physique, most animals run faster than we do, are more graceful (unless we master the torture of the ballet or the sheer exhaustion of the runner). Against the elements we are cosseted, endure heat and cold complaining, have a faculty for soiling our environment unless we contrive disposal systems; we have developed speech and writing yet suffer greatly through ignorance, we are unjust to the weaker and exploit one another on a gigantic scale. We are killers of our kind and then not to eat; we kill for any or no reason at all.

Surely there must be some reason for the duality of our natures which also shows us that we are capable of giving our lives for others, will die readily for our countries even when unaware of the true nature of the conflict. We permit ourselves to be taxed, seldom knowing where the money goes, are educated at great expense and toil in tasks we dislike, develop families which splinter at predictable times, choose our rulers (if choose is the word) for every reason save high morality, ethical excellence, charity of mind, tolerance and wisdom.

Having all of the foregoing qualities and many more, we also bring forth great music and great art, great liars and great frauds. Would even a fox cheat another fox; would even a serpent beat another serpent? Yet we express sublime poetry, drama and the other arts, and when all is done we fear to die—for Nothing in the great beyond.

All of this is known and done to what end? Some religions assert but do not demonstrate that all is in obedience to a creed evolved long ago, of doubtful sense and reason. I believe all are entitled to know that life continues beyond death. The reason for the emergence of spirit healing, then, is this: no other service could more wisely instruct mankind in the truths of his being and potential as do the facts and truths revealed in healing when fully applied and understood in their wide implications.

Spirit healing declares the whole nature, inner and outer, the flesh and the spirit. As we are inwardly, so are we outwardly—an ancient truth.

The physical wonders of man are but a muted metaphor of the spirit self, when we regard the marvels of flow and effect, of the electric responses, the harmony of the healed nature and the beauty of the soul at peace within—by bright eye, tone of voice, rhythm of step, and taken all in all, a wonder of wonders.

Can the mould be less than the casting thrown from the mould, made by beings even wonderful beyond man? If man the model is greater than spirit the designer, then we are indeed all apparitions, having neither tongue nor mind, nor step nor glance, nor love nor compassion. Man may not be the measure of all things but much that is beyond man is foreshadowed by man himself, for he is godlike in his becoming, hence his errant ways for a lesson, for a moulding, for a refining, for a spiritualising.

In spirit healing man comes close to the source of life, guided by those who go before him to mark the way. A day will come when we will see more wonderful things than before. In that day we will be at peace, nation to nation, sex to sex, groups and the alone, all unafraid to live day by day because they will know tomorrow is endless and revealing of good.

Such concepts as are now arising generally in the minds of the thought-shapers would not have been born but for those who have beaten the paths with bleeding feet upon the rocky roads to liberation. There is no need for fear since we cannot, as spirits, be destroyed. The cynics will mock, crying death is death. The knower will sing, death is but a note in the symphony of life. But for the evidence of Survival and its witness, but for the compassionate service called healing, the sacrifices of myriads of unknown pioneers and martyrs would have been all for nothing.

It is a great age to be alive in. It is a great challenge to those whose understanding trembles with joyful anticipation that even in a world of uncertainties, there is a guarantee of a better, fairer, juster, more compassionate world because so many can affirm from their souls' conviction that we are all, without exception, on the road to freedom no matter how long we tarry on the way.

As one closely identified with Spiritualism and with spirit healing and with certain spirit guides. I can say that the healers in the spirit world do not appear to be eager to disclose information as to the energies involved beyond this:

That all kinds of scientists, doctors and others in the

spirit world are involved, that research there is at least as continuous as it is here.

That changes and progress are unending and that no way has yet been found to disclose the keys to a knowledge of the source, nature and application of spirit healing.

That the healer/medium is an indispensable unit in the process of healing.

That the spiritual, mental, psychic and physical development of the healer/medium are factors in the "healing mix" of forces.

That the existence of like factors in the person to be healed are contributory to the healing.

That the human views of the morality, beliefs and so on of the sufferer are not decisive, or even important.

That the "appropriate mix" is the deciding factor, coupled with the circumstances of the occasion, and that maintaining the healed condition is a duty the healed one has to carry out.

That there is not yet a reason given by healers in the spirit for success, partial success or failure.

These views are apparently the best we can produce at this point in development.

In returning to the Dr. Smith experiment on distressed seeds, wounded mice and magnetism, it should be noted that not at any point did the experimenters look beyond the healer to the healing as furnishing evidence either of "outside" influence, change of personality, "split personality", or any of the many variations offered by psychologists, psychic researchers and other unclassified experts. Why? Would not the experiments have been decisive? Did Mr. E know the secret of the energies? The reports are silent; the results speak out clearly.

Then comes the incident of Mr. E's healing, at the request of a hospital chief of staff, of a woman "clinically at the point of death". Two healings, and she was discharged, presumably alive. Why did not Dr. Smith, and others, speculate on the cause of that healing? The diagnosis seemed clear; so was the healing. Yet, no theory, as in the case of the mice, the seeds, the magnetic forces.

The conclusion must then be that scientific research long continued seems to beget only more such research; that until some thoughtful persons beyond, our outside science, make basic discoveries in this field, there will not be scientific progress beyond the present limitations.

The more progressive scientist has to ask: why? Upon the answer much will depend—for science. For the rest of us, healing, spirit healing will develop as forecast.

Another question should have been asked: what is the function of the healer in the act of healing? The best answer I have received so far is: the healer is the catalyst of the forces directed from the spirit state of consciousness to the earthly human consciousness. The catalyst is used to produce change in energy but remains itself unchanged. Yet, even there, and the explanation is from a spirit with much experience, there is room for discussion in this direction: The medium/healer cannot avoid being modified in consciousness as a result of healing. What the change amounts to is a different question. There is one physical analogy we may consider: Electrical energy is transformed down to a level at which it may be used variously since it cannot be used, say, in a household at the pressure reached at the generating station. Whether there are other changes, chemical or atomic, in the act of healing I do not yet have information, although speculation would say there are changes.

I am forced to return to Mr. E's healing of the dying woman:

Are scientific researchers in general more interested in wholly physical manifestations of unknown psychic energies, and do they choose to refuse to look beyond the phenomena, no matter how fascinating, to the cause or causes and, more important, to the implications of the phenomena?

It is a speculation on the attitude of the scientist: is a human being less interesting than a nameless force activating a test instrument. Are the instruments and statistics more attractive than people?

As to the spirit-directed phenomena cited earlier in the science section being evidence for human existence beyond death, it was designated to arouse attention and generate controversy. The period of agitating the scientific and the lay mind was distinguished by the high evidentiality of the phenomena, by the persistence and unfairness of the attacks, and even the bitter and unscrupulous disregard for the safety of the mediums concerned.

Another feature was the widespread character of the Spiritualist movement as the principal source of phenomena, a character that has not diminished but increased.

One more point: As the public mind became more sympathetic to claims for evidence of Survival, new aspects of mediumship were developed until today that gift is, on occasion, publicly displayed on television. While the claims of orthodox churches continue to attract fewer and fewer adherents, the claims of Spiritualism increasingly attract. There is a message here also for physical science—that it should not be afraid to face frankly the paradox developed by such incidents as are dealt with in this postscript.

To the reflective mind the preceding observations should have presented many questions beyond the scope of these notes such as: If what is said be true, why has so little been done? The answer is that much has been and is being done, the ending of the fear of death being one, the availability of healing is another and the spread of a new philosophy of life is another. Can any church offer so much? Can even science offer so much? The answer is no.

Cancer: Revolt of the Cells

Healthy Cells Mean Healthy People

Frustrations Lead to Cancer

Why Women More Affected by Cancer

How Can Cancer be Prevented?

Psychic Nature Bridge Between Physical and Spiritual

The Healing Intelligence

Archbishop's Commission

Doctors Ignore Evidence

## THE CANCER STORY

From the cellular to the celestial is a long journey on our way to deeper understanding of the human unit and of spirit healing. Much has become known of the nature and function of the cell since the basic theory of its structure was developed in the mid-19th century by two German scientists. It is significant that the cell's role in our lives began to be known in the same time span covering the emergence of early, modern knowledge of the human psychic nature. As with other developments, knowledge of cellular activity emerged in the same era as did Spiritualism and other significant discoveries; more signposts to greater revelation were being passed.

Today the general view is that all living bodies are composed of cells. The word "living" is borrowed from a textbook on biology I am consulting now. How can there be anything "non-living"? Discovery of the cell's role in our lives should have led to the view that all life is one, divisible only as we choose to make separations based upon unexplained origin and known by structure and function. Biologists say: "at first the cell's origin was obscure", meaning nobody knew. Later it became clearer: "We now know that all cells result from division of pre-existing cells but for many years it was thought cells might arise more or less spontaneously from non-living material." That concept died, struggling.

The physical concept of "spontaneous" as a scientific explanation, or theory, of a natural phenomenon fails, since it obscures thought by not meeting scientific requirements. It is not demonstrable that any natural phenomenon arises from itself, by internal force or tendency, without direct cause. If this were so we would have to face the question: "Are phenomena self-creating?" "Self-creation or generation" is a misnomer for "we do not know". This is true not only in physical science but in the science and art of spirit healing. There we have discovered only part of the means or methods of transmitting psychic and/or spiritual forces or energies from one state to another or others. How? It seems to operate by reason of the superior position from which spirits operate. Unless they possess or exert powers superior to ours then they are not, in the healing sense, superior. You could argue and ask, are they superior in all or some other matters? The questions are excellent. I do not have the answers, save that the massive healings proved as being of spirit origin place the healers in the spirit in a position superior to ours. Here is no "spontaneous" healing. Here is no "it just happened" explanation. You may argue a causeless cause or random chance but the evidence is against it for reasons all based upon experiences millions of times repeated.

This is not intended as a handy guide to biology (for which I have no qualification) or a dissertation on cells save as they are basic to the body, little understood by laymen, and when researched by specialists disclose facts and functions which all move in a synthesis, exploring and, to me, explaining part, at least, the application of healing power from the spirit realm through healer/mediums to the relief of human disease and suffering.

Spirit healing, at the point of application, is an art since the mediums do not know how to handle the power, or force, or energy. The art consists of the healers making themselves available through attunement for development out of compassion and because their inner natures so prompt them. This still does not amount to knowing how to apply the unnamed power to a specific condition.

This does not deny that through experience the healer/medium becomes more attuned to the healing spirits and in time acquires increasing understanding of the process for which he is a channel. Long and close association leads to acquisition of awareness of what is done. The healer, a living, growing intelligence, takes on some of the characteristics of the spirit guide through continuing co-operation and communication. From the healing service rendered the healer/medium gains increasing sensitivity to the healing spirits until, in some cases, the relationship becomes so close that only those who are familiar with the mediums can note the difference of personality and characteristics.

From personal experience I know this to be so with other mediums. I reason that if this is so for me—then it must be so for others like me, even taking into account the fact that each healer is a distinct entity, with a unique heredity, a unique psychic and spiritual nature. Only highly evolved human beings can direct and influence such sensitive instruments. The task is beyond us. It is a separate study in the subject of spirit science and art.

These considerations are part of the development of an overall view to be stated in a necessary summation. This much is sure: we witness the onset of sweeping changes in all human affairs. The causes are not hard to find. The purpose of the changes is clear to some. Humanity looks for assurance of improvement, for peace within and without, and with a demonstrated, reasoned case for a spiritualised world.

There are criticisms made by those who think the spirit guides do not provide sufficient information on curing diseases. This implies a desire to know in order to be able to do. That information, it is explained, is, so far, beyond our understanding. But, enough is now known so that the healing mission spreads until most of us are aware of the general case.

The statements made here as to the processes in healing cancer are given from a spirit source to Edwards. These views are fully set out in his brochure on cancer where there is a full explanation of the processes whereby a normal, disciplined cell is changed into a malignant, undisciplined cell which runs amok and triggers development of the cancer tumour.

For nearly a century cancer researchers have sought in vain an explanation of those processes. They will, because of their rigid views, continue to ignore the weight and worth of the spirit explanation because it is unorthodox and cannot be discerned under the microscope, since the cause is beyond the scope of the microscope.

Cells enlarged to more than a million times their actual size are shown on British and American TV. Since healing is directed at cells in at least one phase of treatment it may help us realise how intricate and complex and delicately we are harmonised. Being so carefully orchestrated we should learn how to think, feel and act so that the harmonic balance is maintained in such condition that we do not cause a breakdown in any bodily system—no matter which one, or any combination we consider, whether it be the brain, the vision, movement, respiration, sleep, digestion and so on. We cannot hope to hold in our minds at all times every system, every electrical discharge, but we can, if we choose, by effort of will and by patient discipline produce harmony of spirit, mind and body, with the spirit as composer of our music of life.

The mind, in turn, will faithfully transmit all orders and effects to the appropriate glands which, in turn, will carry the news to each organism or group of organisms, down to the cells and beyond. At that level we are close to the essence of harmony. Certain thoughts, feelings and acts will produce certain responses. If we overload, say, the vision system it will endeavour to make a correction. Overloading long continued will produce loss of clarity in the other factors of vision. And so on throughout the whole dazzling array of organs and organisms.

By extending this concept to a long period of overloading we will certainly lose power in each unit so mistreated. The cell that was shown magnified one million times was seen by many TV viewers as a living entity, with reproductive and other systems in action. Any cell also has its nucleus, as an atom does, and contains chromosomes which contain the genes that carry the formative force called heredity: the matrix we bring by birth. It is as though the cell, from one viewpoint, is also a bank or reservoir which handles all kinds of influences in perfect order, whether they are the results of acts, thoughts and emotions beneficial or harmful to us. If we live close enough to the kind of life that is free from fear, greed, hate or any other harmful outlook we can almost surely look for a health harmony—unless we bring into birth a matrix stamped with the imprint of a heredity that requires much modification as well as much development.

We can and do modify heredity by our influence upon the control glands and upon the genes. How else can we change? Do we require an unending series of lives to work out every flaw in our natures? I think not and that even in one lifetime of thoughtful self-discipline—and selfless service—we can, in effect, carry out a peaceful and successful revolution within our own natures. Having achieved so much, we are the better equipped to heal and teach others so that the burden of sickness and ignorance may be, by that much, reduced. And so, from one to many.

This is part of the matrix, expressed through the genes we bring with us into this life. It is not an unyielding metal but a spirit pattern; it changes as we develop.

There is much more to the structure and function of a single cell with its chromosomes that carry the genes, themselves carriers, or seeds, of heredity. These genes are modified and influenced by the motivation of our lives. Everything in the whole human organism responds to everything we do and are. The cell is our inner world expressed in terms beyond the power of microscopes. We cannot escape the consequences of our directives. Nothing is hidden from our supersensitive systems; all is a unity, which is a lesson for us as responsible souls. Therefore, as we become so does our society and the world become. There is no escape.

The cells but respond as we act under the direction of our conscience, do the right deed, feel the right emotions, think the right thoughts. Then, what is right? Right is that which maintains the marvellous human being in harmony—no fear, no anger, no hatred, no jealousy, no envy. Anyone can extend the list: we each know in our hearts how we should live. We do not always know the justice of the condition we have each developed when we seek healing; but our plea is its own message.

You have already read of the healer who healed distressed seeds. That is an instance of cellular healing. And the case of the helpless wounded mice, and of the woman at the point of death.

Highly enlarged displays of a cell or cells under a microscope supports the statement received from spirit that cells are sensitive units of life as everything is sensitive and that, for example, the disease of cancer proceeds from adverse living. Cells are divided into two groups:

1. Those which control and direct physical needs,

2. Those which respond to our thoughts. These latter, says Edwards, are prone to cancer.

In support of that view Edwards cites a study of women with breast cancer. In each case "the normal purposes and functions of a woman's life were frustrated". He reasons that frustration stemming from lack of child-bearing adversely affects the cells most closely related to child-bearing—mainly in the breasts and ovaries. Edwards notes other frustrations arising from absence of child-bearing. In men, problems such as lack of sexual satisfaction led to cancer of the testes "or when a man has endured a harrowing life with much responsibility, causing over-concern with his schemes of life, cancer may arise in the abdomen—which is but an extension of the cause of gastric ulcers".

So, when the genes are adversely influenced, organic harmony is disrupted and we are sick. Cellular reproduction weakness develops and the natural drive of the cells is thwarted. Weakened glands loosen control of the cells which run wild in their capacity to reproduce.

Revolt by one cell spreads, the sick ones preying upon the healthy; a microcosm of the anarchy in societies misled by human beings unbalanced by hate and the desire to dominate.

The immediate causes of cancer differ in each person, Edwards suggests, and evidence supports, the view that since we each have different life motivations, we tend to produce different frustrations in our cells which are reflected in cellular behaviour.

Frustration is a primary cause of cellular disharmony arising from the failure to achieve a "life directive", for example, the desire of a woman for a baby, or other deep mental and emotional distress.

Edwards has positive views on cancer prevention. Considering his vast healing experience his views command respect and attention. We discussed this question at length. I argued that frustration alone could not be the sole cause of cancer, citing my own life as a record of frustration and that frustration is a way of life for most of us. Edwards responded that I must have had some counter-balancing experiences and that awareness of spirit influence and co-operation with it could have maintained the bodily harmony.

We also discussed cancer-causing work conditions. His view is that genetic predisposition is at the root of the cause, augmented by frustration and adverse environment, including domestic and other relationships.

The cellular revolt that is cancer begins with the individual cell. This cell develops a condition of imbalance, "loses its head", so to speak. Unless controlled or reversed to its normally balanced or healthy condition, a tumour, benign or malign develops.

The single, unbalanced cell, in its condition of revolt, adversely affects other cells. There is some recent scientific information to support that fact, since it has been found that "contaminated" cells devour other cells.

The dominant, unbalanced, cell is no different from the unbalanced, mad dictator who, being insane, spreads insanity among his people with consequences we all have experienced. In essence, the cell and the nation are reflections of one another.

The benign tumour can be reversed into a healthy condition, as has been done, by spirit healing in which spirit beings of advanced knowledge direct non-physical energies into bodily conditions which are changed chemically into healthy conditions.

The malign tumour can be healed by the same science and art and health, or harmony, is restored. The cure itself is not merely a touch, it is the application of a superior forces or energies, the first of which is an awareness of peace—the revolt of the mad cells has been halted, and the healing begun.

On reflection I share his conviction not only because of his superior knowledge but also for the following reasons: That we do not yet know the point at which genetic upset involving a cellular rebellion occurs, nor do we know how often we change our motivation in such a positive and beneficial manner that harmony returns and healing of the cells develops.

Many people are cancer-prone. When healing is given the wise influence exercised by spirit guardians changes the outlook and overcomes the birth of the cancer cell. Although there is not yet clear evidence, there is a reason to believe, through experience, that many have been spared the onset of cancer through the influence of spirit healing.

If this is so, then spirit healing is an adjunct and not a way of life. In case I am faced with any orthodoxy in healing and in Spiritualism, the answer is that we are all free to speculate and all may err—and some succeed. This much must be said; all efforts at self-control leading hopefully towards a state of peace within will fail unless we learn—until it becomes second nature—to be as healers should be when they serve—serene, ready to give.

If we can, in time, and after many failures arrive at such a habit of non-tension then we may discover we are on the way to that condition in life where we need not seek healing but are become healers, that is, as a light to others in darkness and as a haven where troubled souls may find peace and guidance.

Much that is written by Edwards, by me and by others may surprise the newcomer to healing since the common response to mention of the subject is, "Oh, faith healing". When that is dealt with, the next approach is, "Oh, laying on hands". There is so much to be told, so much to be learned that we may only report what we know and speculate that, with the years, we will know more and do better.

Since we cannot look to scientists for co-operation in seeking greater knowledge of spirit healing we must continue as we began: by trial and inspiration, a justifiable alternative. At this point I will try to resume the thread of a progressive mission expressed through, first, evidence of Survival, by a wide range of evidence, and second, a healing mission. The evidential battle is won. The healing mission is established and like a successful army that has breached a line of defence, fans out for complete victory. It is so easy for me to write "the healing mission is established"; yet it is so. Before racing on to claim triumph, we should look around a little.

What is intended now is a survey of the road we have come. From there we can attempt the venture that has disproved so many prophecies. Frankness may persuade where eloquence fails. By what authority do we say there is a spirit-inspired, spirit-directed, evidentiary, healing and teaching mission? By the following:

Of all the movements in the past 150 years or so where there have been signs of spirit co-operation, only one movement has openly and courageously maintained contact with those spirit guides and others in the spirit world who are concerned not only with communication but with the regeneration of man. This is not to claim we are better than others, know more than others, therefore, should be heard with deference. Our only claim upon public attention is that we have kept our compact with those who rely upon us to serve always, to be faithful to what we know to be true, to refuse to submit to attacks, threats and misrepresentation. We have so served to a persuasive degree or we would not now be in our present position as the only group in the world teaching and demonstrating without respite that man is a spiritual being and that from such truth flows much that he needs to know.

From such loyalty to service the healing mission grew

and grows daily, while the evidence-producing service is also increasing. I do not mean to derogate any other organisation by stating that we succeed (if that is the word) while others are falling away. The evidence for our continued growth, with little or no organisation, is in the numbers given proof of Survival and healing. To have so influenced millions without a priesthood, without schools of theology, with limited resources is, to me, evidence that there is a non-physical support. Of this I am sure because the evidence is overwhelming in my life and the lives of my friends and contemporaries.

We have already seen that physical science, through its most eminent thinkers, accepts the view that thought is the "ultimate" ground upon which it now stands; it formerly was matter that was the "ultimate". It took scientists centuries to move from matter to thought although no scientist has yet seen a thought, or weighed or measured, or touched a thought, yet they now theorise its ultimate reality.

Spirit counsellors say thought may by us be regarded as an energy formation perceived by the mind, then transmitted to the computer brain of man and recognisable to the recipient. By reproducing their thoughts in the minds of others, they have shown they can reproduce and influence others, that is, spirits in the flesh. Thought is a definite energy in a distinct, characterised form, that is, it has its own character or personality. This is how spirit doctors guide and help patients who are under mental stress. That is a description of part of the process of mental healing. This shows that the healers in spirit use a method of conveying a thought to a mind capable of receiving it.

This not only throws light upon an aspect of spiritual healing but leads us to wider, deeper views of inspiration, original thoughts. It is one more evidence of the revolution in our thinking developed from the Science and Art of Healing; it explains how men and women of limited education do, in time, develop or receive ideas surpassing the rigidities of the orthodox. Indeed, Spiritual Healing is the Science and Art of the Soul which has only begun to enlighten mankind of greater things to follow.

It is not difficult to accept, after analysis based upon some kind of experience, the view that this world, physically material as it is said to be, is based upon thought, the invisible matrix of all matter. This, granted as a premise, we next say: do atoms and cells fall within the same category? No, the atom, an organisation of energy, is not seen, but is measured. The cell may be seen microscopically. By gradation we see that the road to accepting invisible thought is not so rough.

The mind (already shown not to be the brain) is the king in our bodies, yet it is disembodied. Where does it live? Does it have points of contact with the brain, the skin and so on? We do not know that, but we do know the mind is man's organ for dealing with the psychic or dynamic substance, or the mental substance, called thought. It could be that ectoplasm is a physical version of thought. Thought, as metaphysical substance, produces ideas. Ideas are created by necessity. We ask: Then what is will? The answer has to be: the desire and purpose which gives form to thought, emotion and action.

Are we, as thinking souls, like all other organisms, capable of creating ideas out of thought by direction of the will? Then, having gone so far, we may say that imagination is shown by the images into which it is cast by the will. This takes us into the concept that we shape ideas from a psychic substance called thought and direct these ideas by will. That seems to be a tidy, complete statement. How do we demonstrate it?

Can we take pictures of thoughts and of spirit people?

I have already so testified. The pictures referred to are on file in the *Psychic News* library in London. There must be thousands of psychic pictures all over England. Some of the "thought pictures" referred to were produced during a two-city experiment in thought transference—or what is called telepathy. My own experience is conclusive to me. Others have wider experience. (As I write this I have on the table a spirit picture of W. T. Stead, famous editor and medium. The likeness was impressed on a plate I held while Arthur Ford identified the spirit. I also heard a band play the hymn "Nearer My God to Thee". Stead went down on the *Titanic*. Before I left London he said he would be with me.)

A Japanese, Prof. Fukurai, wrote and illustrated a book titled *Thoughtography*. It dealt with pictures he had taken of a Japanese medium projecting thoughts. Many contemporary researchers are excited by special camera work showing a variety of non-physical shapes. Is an idea a shape of thought? If so, who or what shapes the thought into an idea?

We are not talking about miracles (that is, phenomena said to be caused by magic or its equivalent, the spontaneous) but about the phenomena upon which our individual lives are based. Remove the normally invisible thoughts, ideas and emotions and we have little left, maybe the instincts or automatic responses of the body. Take away invisible, intangible, weightless, soundless mind—and what have we got? Mindless we are nothing. With mind we are creators. Then, is mind everywhere? Genes and cells have minds. Cells are remarkable people, in a way.

The mind as creator may be directed by the will of the human spirit, in or out of the flesh. In the flesh, there are many limitations.

Beyond, and with the flesh, we co-operate with the liberated spirits across the psychic bridge and all the rest follows which brings us to the role of the mind in spirit healing—which is also intelligent, invisible, silent and creative. Strange is it not that we live by the unseen yet deny the reality of the phenomena it produces as a reflection of itself?

Anyone may become an expert in the religion of the mind, which means that view of life which regards mind as another expression of life meaning "God as Mind". Some movements are based upon that concept, especially in America. In the Orient it has been commonplace for centuries. Yet all of this leads us to our main goal which is to state the most we know and theorise about spirit healing which is, finally, a Spirit Science, and we may yet discover it is The Spirit Science and the root of the science of life.

We can not be mentally serene unless we have a compelling reason for such an attitude. The man awaiting execution is not a good subject for instruction in the benefits of serenity. The mind afraid is not easily pacified, and so on. In healing there has to be a reciprocity between our minds and the minds of those who from another sphere direct such force or power as will restore the harmony in the body which we have lost by fear or any other self-destroying thoughts—all of which come from the mind.

Spirit healing restores harmony by wise influence and guidance. The balanced mind sets the restorative patterns for the legions of cells and so on within the body—and we are again in harmony. All of this should persuade we erring humans that what we call peace of mind should be an integrated aspect of our lives, more important than any other activity apart from those we must undertake to meet our responsibilities.

The aim and purpose of setting out a case for the reality and primacy of the mind is to show how we must deal with our own natures so that we evolve as was designed. If we were not in the age when such counsel is made available we would be in a worse position than we are now. By the exertions of pioneers whose names are lost to us we are now so placed that we live in a climate of thought less hostile to views such as ours than at any other time of record. We do think and speculate freely—surely an activity of the mind.

It is not by mere happenstance that interest in the psychic world alone has grown so great; there is an equal, if not greater, pressure for instruction in matters spiritual. Much that a century ago was regarded as mystery is now made clear and explained by factual information that a citizen of that time returning to this earth now would not grasp the difference. We learn daily that mind functions at all levels, within our consciousness, and that we learn through the impact of thoughts from other minds, incarnate and discarnate, whether we are aware of the process or not.

Because we are spirits we can receive spirit healing. There is no other way. The more we develop our spiritual natures the more readily do intimations of the spirit impinge on our consciousness. Like calls to like. This is the change wrought by the efforts of the army of nameless pioneers. This has brought us to the question posed in a paraphrase of a biblical text dealing with spirit communication: "Try them to see if they are of God" and additionally we are asked to see with what bodies they come. The first injunction is easily understood; the second requires much explanation since the author of that biblical statement was clearly a well-informed medium who asked more questions than he answered.

In his writing on the healing intelligence Edwards confirms now what students of the occult and oriental teaching have been saying for many years: that the pituitary gland is the most important ductless gland in the body, with an increasing number of functions being attributed to it—including influence over all other glands, by disciplining cells, governing the sexual systems, "and that it operates without the need for direct orders from the mind or brain; thus it possesses an individual intelligence". Occultists say it is the pineal gland which is the direct link between the spirit and the body consciousness. Therefore, we may claim that this small marvellous organ plays a major role in communication between souls in the body and those in the spirit; also it may be the control centre through which spirit healing power moves swift as thought to bodily areas and that responses race back to the mind.

Already we have the view of an eminent neurologist that the human brain far exceeds the capability of any computer. The brain is the servant of the mind and is the directing centre for all bodily functions—an amazing complex. The mind retrieves through the brain all stored information required to deal with life's unending situations. Each unit of the human cosmos has its function; each reports continuously; decisions are made at speeds baffling to laymen, yet when we fall ill we complain. How should nature complain? The body and the mind and the soul should complain; the harmony has been blocked. Their complaints have the shape and sound called disease.

The foregoing is, in part, a summary of a portion of Edwards' excellent book, *The Healing Intelligence*, which should become the classic work on the role of the mind in healing. It is a profound experience and has no equal in any lay literature because Edwards has successfully devoted a lifetime to the healing arts and has laid the foundation for a human version of the healing science and art. All of this is done because as an instrument of the spirit he has absorbed much knowledge: payment for service rendered. He is not the "automaton" mediums are supposed to be.

The occultists say there is a close connection between the pineal gland and the pituitary gland as links between the body and the spirit. Edwards' views—and mine—are that they are as stated, the communication centres, back and forth, from soul to psychic nature, to body and back again as long as the soul can maintain its hold upon the body—its empire for experience on earth.

In studying the statements just made it becomes easier to accept the now recognised view that much disease develops from what is here called soul sickness—the psychosomatic. When the claims made as to the functions of the pineal and pituitary glands are analysed it is clear that the bodily systems are so sensitive in their responses to all stimuli that we can no longer resist the case for their role in our lives.

Let us not pause to elaborate on the occult literature on this point save to say that the pineal and the pituitary still have a vital role in the human body. For the pituitary the role of secreting hormones is medically established. It is a speculation on my part that these two organs, the pineal and pituitary, are currently increasing their influence on psychics in this period of increasing awareness of our inner natures. Increasing exercise of psychic and spiritual gifts is a direct response to the influences from the spirit world. As we awaken to spirit influence it is because the pineal and pituitary are stimulated by our spirit teachers and guides. It is a reasonable view that for increased receptivity we require increased capacity. Again the two-way exchanges.

Consider this: as an outstanding example Edwards has developed to a pre-eminent point as a spirit healer. Why Edwards? Because, apart from other things, he is of such a psychic and spiritual nature and was possessed from birth (or before) with such specific innate capabilities that he had only to be stimulated to achieve his successes as a healer—and author. As he began he was unaware of all of this. Again the power was not under his control. As he served knowledge flowed into his consciousness as water flows downhill. Increased knowledge brought increased capacity to receive new concepts which had to move from spirit teachers and healers to his mind by way of the pineal and the pituitary to his brain consciousness. These, the pineal and the pituitary, increased in capacity as their natural, prehistoric functions were renewed. Only in such men (and women) may such gifts as spirit healing and other faculties be brought to a high pitch of beneficial use. It is as though sleeping giants awakened, except that the two giants are so small as not to warrant close scientific attention in studies of the psychic and spiritual nature.

I believe we have entered a period of increasing stimulation by the inner world of our psychic and spiritual gifts. The stimulation always originates there. It becomes manifest here in a variety of phenomenal forms.

Since these two centres, or sentinels, the pineal and the pituitary, stand guard at the doors of consciousness they relay thoughts and other forces from the physical to the spiritual. When all has been analysed in time so fleeting swift as to be immeasurable the answers and directions flash back to the sentinels by way of the mind to the brain by way of the little giants—and we become aware.

In viewing just two functions, the cellular and the cerebral, we are justified in pausing to marvel that we are so made and yet so wantonly misuse our bodies as to fall ill. Even there we have a plea in mitigation of our offences against the self since often we are helpless against the forces of society. When our lives are endured in poverty, dirt, disease, hunger and in want of spiritual nourishment, is it any wonder that we become prey to what are called the psychosomatic illnesses? That long

Latin word means soul sickness. We know the condition if we cannot give the definition. Indeed, nature has no definitions; we coin them to be reminded of their existence.

The line of cause and effect: Fear the cause, cancer the eventual effect, is now, medically, more openly recognised by orthodox medicine. Without listing the common ailments of mankind it is easy to see that what is demonstrated in one case will apply to others—whether they be cancer or any other disease. The principle once established, the complications follow.

That is the scientific aspect: Knowing.

Now we come to the Art of Healing: Doing.

Assuming that the foregoing views are valid as to the cause of a disease (influence of the mind and emotions) what are the facts in applying spirit healing?

The answer is that there is a reverse process: by thought and will psychic and/or spirit energies are brought to bear on the bodily conditions. These energies strengthen the now weakened cellular and other structures so that natural processes are brought up to the level of efficiency required to maintain that area of the body in a healthy state. In short, the bodily systems weakened by heredity, environment, misuse and the stresses that together produce sickness are strengthened—the outcome is a healing. That is my description of applying knowledge (science) to specific conditions (an art) in order to produce healing. The art lies with the intelligence, which chooses, adapts to changes and finally achieves its objective—healing.

The intelligence of the healer in the spirit is shown in the use of energies whose character and effect must be known, else there would be chaos and the "accidents" that arise from ignorant misuse of powers would not be understood. In spirit healing we have power applied by knowledge—to the benefit of now many millions over the past 130 years at least. Who may figure how many more millions to come? External irritations and other cancer-causing substances do not yet appear to be the indisputable begetters of cancer.

Here is one example out of many cases; taken from Edwards' book, *The Healing Intelligence*, to stimulate discussion:

A form of chronic leukemia (cancer of the blood) was found in a 7-year-old boy in a London hospital. His leukemia was of a kind seen rarely in children. Parents were told by the specialist in charge there was no hope of recovery; deep ray treatment was ruled out. The doctor in charge said if the patient were his son he would not hurt him with that therapy. The official diagnosis was: "chronic myeloid leucosis".

One day later Edwards was asked, by telephone, to give spiritual absent healing to the boy. That was begun immediately. The next day the specialist in the case told the boy's father that an unexplained difference had occurred in the child's condition. From then onwards the boy's blood count improved markedly. This improvement continued so far that the boy was soon sent home and in about three months made a complete recovery. His blood count was normal: he was back in school and active in sports.

The medical view was that the period of improvement would last not more than two years, at most. Edwards writes that seven years later the boy was "well". The family moved. The healer lost contact with the family. Some time later he learned the boy had lived on for nine years more. Edwards did not learn the cause of death. This the healer finds strange because of the way the boy had responded to spirit healing where the specialist said there was no hope of recovery. The parents had then sought the healing and the boy was cured.

At no time did Edwards see the boy.

This case is given because of the recovery in face of the positive medical diagnosis.

It is well worth our time to consider this case because of the light it throws not only on this situation but on other cases, showing how the science and art of healing has operated through more than 15,000,000 cases since the beginning of the Edwards healing mission. He gives this analysis:

The boy was said by a medical specialist to be incurable.

Recovery began within 24 hours of the request, by telephone, for healing.

Since there was no physical contact between the boy and the healer the creative energy must have been directed by an intelligence, one knowing how to apply the energy.

Source of the healing was not physical.

No physical mind has such a capability to heal or it would have been known long since.

Source of the healing was spiritual since it was not physical.

There must have been a harmony between the boy's nature and the spirit nature or he could not have received healing from the spirit source.

The spirit intelligence responsible for the healing must have been able to diagnose accurately, must have known the nature of the disease and must have known how best to apply specific energy or energies to change a diseased condition into a healthy state.

Then there is the matter of knowing how to develop a healthy cellular condition within the body, with each cell having its individuality. In a sense spirit healing gives "first aid" to the healing process so that in the cells their natural, healthy state can be restored. Similarly, the blood chemistry is brought into line with other healing processes, the boy's condition is improved—and healing is proved by his return to school.

Edwards deals, in his analysis, with the step by step development of the healing, presenting a reasoned view of what is involved—a knowledge of biological processes, all under the intelligent direction of an invisible healing spirit or spirits.

He concludes with the declaration already made elsewhere: the transformation from sickness to health occurs when the spirit overshadows the physical self, truly a wonder and mystery beyond our rational understanding. Once the healing is evoked and all systems work towards healing, the spirit intelligence withdraws and the former sufferer is once more responsible for all that occurs. He is once again master in his own house, the body.

The case of the boy recovered from chronic leukemia was one of several submitted to the Commission on Divine Healing set up by the Archbishops of Canterbury and York. Full of prestige? As you will see, also full of prejudice, at the highest level. It is presumptuous, of course, that the Church of England, or any other church, should set itself up as judge of what is and what is not healing, divine or any other. The church has no skill, no experience in the matter, no healers and only an assumed authority. Bishops are ordained by other bishops, not by God. What led the Church of England to assume it could be judge? The question answers itself. Healing, spirit healing, has become popular—because many are being healed—outside the church. The Anglican branch of orthodoxy was no doubt being pressed by some of its liberal-minded ministers and members to "do something".

When the above case of chronic leukemia was submitted to the Archbishops' Commission it was referred to a medical committee which did not ask for medical histories, did not question the parents nor see the boy. This display of prejudice is standard medical, ethical and clerical practice where spirit healers are concerned. And this in a church founded upon spirit healing and spirit return of a great healer.

The resistance of doctors and clergymen to the facts of spirit healing is again shown in the following cases:

A man with a painful throat condition lost his voice. Specialists found malignant tissue and arranged for surgery. The patient called Edwards. Absent healing was given. The swelling was reduced, pain vanished, the voice becoming normal. The man consulted the two specialists who had diagnosed his condition. They were impressed, a second biopsy found all traces of cancer had disappeared, the voice was normal, surgery was not required. Their explanation: "Miracle healing". They did not explain that.

Soon afterwards a prominent doctor was researching about 100 cases of spirit healing supplied by Edwards. The doctor contacted the two specialists involved in the case reported above, asking for their explanation of their patient's recovery. This was their, presumably scientifically-based reply: "By a fortunate coincidence the segment of tissue taken for the first biopsy happened to contain all the cancer cells". It is not credible, but that explanation by two medical specialists was published in the *British Medical Journal* of December 7, 1954, without comment, as the explanation of the healing of the cancer they had diagnosed.

It appears now that medical and theological prejudice is a nearly incurable disease. I should not be surprised or shocked at anything. Yet, there is more to show how men of considerable technical knowledge can be, and are, capable of self-induced mental blindness. Sometimes you wonder if the struggle is worth while. But when one formerly hostile person or organisation moves towards tolerance, it is worth while. The same *British Medical Journal* which published the indefensible view of the two specialists in the throat cancer case, later printed an editorial suggesting that "spontaneous" healings should be investigated. Fine, if late, but when the healings are found not to be "spontaneous" (that is, self-generating) what explanation will then be found?

Do you think that even eminent doctors are superstitious? They have to be, else they could not be talking about spontaneous. Spontaneous is miraculous. Miraculous is beyond the law of cause and effect. If I err here, then the whole case for spirit healing has to be reconsidered and another explanation found for what appears to be cause and effect since all other healings come under that law. If it is argued that healings are sometimes of the spirit and sometimes of the spontaneous, where does the healer come in? If spontaneous is an answer, why does not spontaneous heal more often where doctors fail? Can there be by theological or medical decree a suspension of the natural law to permit spontaneous to heal in some cases and not in another? Spontaneous is a medical and theological alibi.

In the world of the rational, spontaneous means: "I do not know" which is a good place to start in search of knowledge. Nothing moves without a mover. The next question is: how, in which circumstances and by whom or what directed: intelligent direction or blind chance? The logic cannot be escaped but for some time doctors and priests will try and try to find new words as cloaks for ignorance. In this case they do not know and should openly say so. Admission of ignorance is a prerequisite to knowledge.

Here is another example of medical "don't want to know". When Edwards gave evidence before the Archbishops' Commission, a TV doctor threw on his table the case papers relating to 70 healings supplied by

Edwards, with medical records, at the commission's request. It is hoped that the TV doctor's medicine is better than his judgment for he declared, of the documents: "This is not worthwhile evidence, for all of these cases could have been spontaneous".

That should be the end of it, but no, Edwards replied that all the cases offered were "recoveries from diseases said to be medically incurable". The TV doctor's reply to that has the ring of the last word: "Too many doctors are diagnosing incurability when it is not so". Is the medical art of diagnosis so weak?

To show that all clerics are not genetically opposed to spirit healing or healer/mediums, Edwards reports that he was offered a position in the Anglican Church—on conditions he, of course, could not accept. At least someone was listening with a half open mind.

No matter how much we may strive to explain healing by means other than the spirit, we fail. If, as the TV doctor exclaimed, too many doctors diagnose illnesses as incurable, then the cure when it is achieved by means other than the medical has to be due to intelligent spirit action.

Since I trust we agree that the spirit is everywhere, then the mind must also be everywhere. Likewise the psychic. This issue is raised because of the careless use of the concept of spontaneous healing. It could arise from instances of healings so rapid that it appears there was indeed a mistaken diagnosis—or an inexplicable cause of the cure.

How do we explain the case of the man with throat cancer? You could argue that it was "spontaneous", in the sense that it was speedy. Surely speed is not to be accepted as a criterion of either presence or absence of basic spirit. Each person is different by degree from all others, therefore, each person responds differently by degree to spirit healing. When we talk of the healing intelligence surely by intelligence we mean organised knowledge consciously applied to a specific condition not available through any other source but the organism of a certain kind of human being called a healer. That healer is a modified entity capable of transmitting specific energy or energies in such a manner as:

1. Either to stimulate bodily organisms into recifying disease conditions by use of the body's consciousness such as boosting the output of healthy cells or other units or,
2. Temporarily maintaining certain functions until the bodily intelligence is well enough to fulfil its own functions.

Since neither time nor distance are factors in healing and that intelligence, direction and conditions are all, it is reasonable to claim that what seems to be a spontaneous cure (that is arising from itself), cannot be demonstrated on the same basis as, say, the healing of someone either by contact or distant treatment. In the latter case, usually spirit healing is sought when orthodox remedies fail. Then we narrow the area to be examined. It is because I regard spirit healing to be an essential study (and service) that these questions are raised, not because there is any doubt as to the reality and value of spirit healing.

Since this is a story and has many personal references, it is appropriate to state here that I view my lifelong convictions as to the basic truths of Spiritualism and healing as being worthy of continuing examination. Always I have sought some valid alternative explanations, some hitherto unexamined concept to show where error lies. So far all I have gathered is more evidence, more experience and an increasing desire never to persuade myself beyond reasonable doubt.

That is the basis for examining the claims of "spontaneous" cure. Let us look at it another way. A person becomes ill. Medical diagnosis says there is a certain condition. This turns out to be mistaken: equally it may be accurate. Medical care is applied. The patient is not cured. Spirit healing is sought. The healer is attuned to the case by his own inner psychic and spiritual development. Within a day or so, or in my own case already quoted, almost immediately there is a complete cure of a condition said by a doctor to be beyond his skill. "It's between the patient and God." Did God intervene?

We never can find the answer. But the healer, Billy Parish, was called. He could not come because of wartime restrictions. Yet I was aware of two white soothing hands where the pain was at the limit of my endurance. That incident has some of the elements of being "spontaneous" (speed and complete cure), but it was initiated by my wife's appeal for help. In other personal situations I have sought spiritual help. There did not appear to be any response. Was the subsequent cure, or relief, denied me, or did the seeming silence (and indifference) convey the message that I must endure alone and leave the explanation to another day and other circumstances? Failures most frequently tell us more than success; all success is based upon what we have learned from prior failures. I suggest that healers, and others, should always be alert to "failures".

One more point: it seems that there is so much to learn about healing with the co-operation of the spirit that we should consider the view that a sick person for whom healing is sought may be himself a healer unaware of the gift. It could be that of himself and subconsciously he has arrested the sickness condition and has proved a favourable condition. This condition then requires the stimulation supplied by the spirit/healer in co-operation with the medium/healer to produce such changes in the body that the curative process is speeded up. In that sense the claim is made that potentially we are all healers and must be since we are all spirits.

This is the theme I desired to reach. I believe this aspect will be studied for these reasons:

The growth of healing, from being done by a few pioneers largely by one method, contact, has developed until today there are many thousands of healers in Britain alone and the movement spreads. Healings take place one way or another. We become sick either by causing or tolerating adverse physical conditions of many kinds, or by tolerating social and personal conditions which produce fears and tensions of such character and intensity that we are unable to release our own healing powers.

There is no point in arguing for the ideal condition: there is none. All we may achieve is steady progress by percentages to the place where we seldom fall sick, seldom develop or permit conditions which result in disease.

The question of spontaneity brought this up because it had to do so. All who heal or desire to heal should ponder these questions. They represent a progressive view, just as Parish and Edwards ushered in a progressive mode of healing when they healed mainly at a distance and in Edwards' case, initiated other reforms in situations that had become static.

It may come to some as a surprise that there is a prospect all human beings can heal, not equally, but universally, since all can hurt. Healing and hurting are two sides of one coin which represents the human spirit in one way.

Surely the fact of the growing army of healers points in that direction. It requires little imagination to foretell the development of healing. Let us try. To do so we must return briefly to the great mission of the Nazarene and his colleagues. They developed healing—and teaching—

on a wide scale. I am among many who hold that but for the healing—and demonstration of Survival—there is no psychic or spiritual basis for religion. Even a cursory reading of the cultures of many times will show there were many creeds and cults but none with the universality of Survival and Healing and Teaching so clearly demonstrated as by the existing medium/healer movement in this very day.

Now we present healing from a different aspect. Before we considered the lines of development and of frustration with all its implications. The frustration was, and is, not only of the spiritual yearnings of mankind; but frustration enforced without hope of remedy or relief. Beneficial changes which modify the social genes must also modify the physical and spirit genes. Society has been drawn into a state of disease. It is this that attracts healing; the sickness attracts the remedy as the magnet attracts iron. The spirit, not always consciously, seeks the better environment for its expression as the cellular and human organisations seek reproduction.

Poets have sung of the unity of mankind, many reformers have shaped idealistic policies for amelioration of the human lot. But, as stated at the outset, frustration through centuries of misuse of life and its energies have brought us to the climax of crises. No philosophy has persuaded men and societies to live as though they were indeed seeking to live more closely according to the spirit. I do not claim that if we all become healers, in our our varying degrees, that heaven, whatever that may be, will come to earth and all our diseases, physical, psychic and spiritual, will vanish from the earth.

But what is said is this: For the first time mankind has as its choice a knowledge of the reality of spirit, has as its choice a knowledge of the reality of spirit, not the church view, but spirit as the basis of life, not of creeds. This spirit reality is so often demonstrated that it has enabled even the credulous and ignorant to accept and pay for vulgarisations of its phenomena for entertainment, about as futile and degrading as the superstitition called witchcraft.

Healing is as universal a truth as survival of bodily death is a universal truth: they speak all languages, concern all in all circumstances and should be available to all who may choose to co-operate, to their own advantage, or continue in their state of unwillingness to be healed.

In his book, *The Healing Intelligence*, Edwards writes (p. 56): "Unfortunately there exists with a considerable number of sick people, a state of healing inertia. The mind and body of the patient have come to accept the ill-condition as habitual." The sickness is established; doctors have said nothing more can be done; the patient must live with it. Of course, the mind and body adjust as they must, until one day a glimmer of energy penetrates the gloom of surrender, healing is sought (the first necessity); there is a revolution in the soul, the psychic nature and, finally, in the body. Even the bodily consciousness may be stirred into self-reform—and the healing takes hold. A miracle? No, a sequential therapy established and applied by spirit art based upon scientifically acquired knowledge.

It is not only through what we call direct spirit healing that all cures are achieved. I came across such cases in a study of homeopathic medicine. Herbalists, Christian Scientist practitioners can report like instances. The differences are of degree, not principle. The homeopathic or the herbal remedy may convey just that combination of energies that correct even cell imbalance and sickness, then the healing process develops. Homeopaths and herbalists also are influenced by spirit healers. But it is significant in the views offered here that healer/mediums who co-operate consciously and regularly with healing guides heal more persons and achieve greater percentages of cures than any others.

I have referred to this elsewhere and say it results from closer co-operation. This is seen in other facets of mediumship, from trance speaking to inspired writing, music and art. The closer we are to our spirit teachers the more they can express themselves, even to percentages nearing 95. No one with experience will claim that even in the most accomplished mediumship there is complete takeover. The instrument always modifies the message to a degree. But from many experiences we gather many evidences. These together with our own mediations and direct experiences complete the picture.

Now, in healing, the situation is somewhat analogous. The healer will always, but not intentionally, modify the energy, save when he or she is asleep and the healing spirits work with least restrictions from the healer/medium's mind. These considerations are taken up in some detail later. When the body sleeps, the soul awakes.

The relevance here to these considerations is that we co-operate to bring awareness of the spirit nature within nature, called by many other names, the silence, the inner self, the haven of the mystic, refuge of the soul and so on. What we do when we withdraw the focus of our minds is to become free to dwell for a spell in our own environment—the spiritual. This, in part, is what is achieved in the development and experience of the healer and of the medium for other services.

It is not difficult to foresee the coming of the age that will be known as the Democracy of the Spirit. The spread of healing is the most recent signpost we have reached pointing in the direction of a Democracy of the Spirit.

Earlier in this section the parallel was drawn between the Nazarene mission of the first century and the spiritualising mission originally developed through several phases of Spiritualism. The aim is to show progression, stage by stage, through all manner of persecution, through all manner of man-made crises until we achieved the situation and condition in which we now find ourselves. Few of us had such views, say, 40 or 45 years ago; we could not because our experience was still in the future. Now we have arrived at what was once the future. Such prophecy is not mysterious.

It is a good question to ask: How can a conviction of, say, Survival beyond the grave or demonstration of spirit healing help to change the human condition for good without hurting anyone? As already said, men and societies live upon the fruits of the mind, even the scientists who peer into the cells or the stars, even the mother nursing her child at the breast. The most refined and the most oppressed of mankind alike live to the music of the mind. All do not hear the same music but they do so live for there is no alternative. When we have such experiences as persuade the thoughtful to realise there is a Beyond and a Within they must obey their minds for it is upon that magnificent instrument, that the harmonies of the soul express what we were, what we have become and what we are becoming.

Once persuade man that he is imperishable, as a spirit, a deathless entity with unending development, surely he will, in time, consider that actions contrary to that truth will work to his disadvantage. He will not be killed for disobedience of the Law of Life, but will retard his own progress by exactly the measure of his wrong-doing to others. And he will advance directly as he lives in healing with all his fellows and with nature.

That view is set out in all basic religious concepts. Spiritualism and its services go farther in demonstrations providing proof, not speculation, that the basic concepts are founded in fact. There is the difference between an arid man-made creed and a religion built upon a Science and Art, as exemplified in spirit healing.

For the reasons stated I foresee a revolution in thought. The human spirits, here and Beyond, have so long engaged in such enterprises as healing and teaching of our inner capabilities that the weight and force of the consequent convictions must change public opinion. Public opinion must, in time, be changed through the effects of the Democracy of Healing. This combined with the scientific evidence of Survival must persuade man that killing the body does not solve our problems and that healing the body—and the mind—provides a foundation for new societies freed from fear either of sickness or death.

When we are persuaded that Life is Continuous we also learn we have potential for power beyond the imagination of all other ages.

So, the wheel comes full circle—from the primitive to the sophisticated; from men huddled before a fire in a forest or seeing shapes in the shadows they cast on the walls of their caves, stirring their imaginations, to the point at which we are now poised: shall we reap the harvests of the centuries of striving, or, shall we continue to kill, exploit, corrupt, mislead and endanger the whole species?

We have, at our command, all the knowledge required to heal our sick world since we know now how to heal, person to person, and become aware that we all travel the same path. We know that, as spirits, we are deathless. What more do we require? More to eat? Together we can provide abundance by applying our knowledge. Do we require knowledge? It can be made available to all without exception. Do we require to travel? The skies offer no barrier. Do we wish to cleanse our air and oceans and rivers? We can do even that by curbing greed, by control of the polluters, not the pollution.

We can end poverty, reduce ignorance, and develop healing to the state where we will cease to manufacture disease because we will cease to provide the emotional and mental conditions which breed disease.

I can hear the cynic: What about pests? Well, what about them? They, surely, can be controlled without our poisoning our soil or water.

Enough has been said to show that we have the required knowledge, physical, mental, psychic and spiritual, to provide the environment at all levels and phases of consciousness to regenerate the world. Shall we?

How Spirit Healers
are Developed

Edwards, Pioneer of
Simplified Healing

Spirit Power
Directed by Spirit
Intelligence

Attunement to Spirit

Key to Spirit Healing

How Spirit Healers
on Earth
Co-operate with
Unseen Healers

## THE ART OF HEALING

Many who desire to heal become attached to a Spiritualist church or other group working on the basis of Spiritualist evidence and teaching. Effectiveness of the teaching methods is always tested by results. In most cases it is difficult to arrive at reasonably accurate figures. Yet, as long as some healing is achieved it matters little that the best-tested methods are not always followed carefully. The reason for advising study and practice at some centre where experienced healers serve is that where healings are more successful healers become more confident. In this way they become more competent, consequently more effective and the healing experience attracts more volunteers.

Under the presidency of Harry Edwards the National Federation of Spiritual Healers has developed to the point that it has more than 8,000 members and as an international organisation will take the healing mission and its methods to many other countries. Edwards, at 81, resigned his post, having brought the organisation—and healing—to a high point of public recognition and acceptance.

The basic training course offered by the National Federation of Spiritual Healers was developed by Edwards based upon his long experience. Teaching covers generally the human anatomy and organic functions, with simplified outlines of cellular and other processes and some scientific information. The brain is clearly described. This is done to provide healers with a background of information so that when healing by the contact or absent method, they can visualise a living group of human systems, working towards that harmony called health.

The simple, step by step, application of spirit healing is set out so that anyone with even a modest education can follow. I advise anyone wishing to become a healer to contact the healers' organisation to obtain, among other things, the correspondence courses. There is no final passing examination but there is a questionnaire to estimate whether the teaching has served its purpose to inform and teach. Also, the results provide material for correcting or improving the courses.

I do not attempt a summary of the valuable courses since that is the function of the National Federation of Spirit Healers, Shortacres, Church Hill, Loughton, Essex. Mr. Gilbert Anderson is the Administrator.

Because of the general lack of knowledge of the "how" of spirit healing, especially by mediums who understand the case for the method, here is a statement of some of the practices formerly followed merely because they had become habits untested by critical examination. Almost all previously followed practices have been challenged and discarded because they had become habits. The tendency to accept the accepted way of doing things is strong and avoids the need to be firm in examination of all methods—old and new.

The laying on of hands in healing is a natural and probably unschooled development arising from the basic desire to communicate by touch, with all of the acts that follow touch or bodily contact. Agreements were, and are, sealed by handshake; "take your hands off me" is a form of rejection, and so on through many variations. Babies are soothed by caressing hands. And many die at the hands of others. The reader can supply his own variation on the theme of "touch me, touch me not". The lore of the hand is vast; in spirit healing it has a place, but not the place.

In keeping with Edwards' views on this and other matters that I share, he gives reasoned counsel on the use and value of the hands in healing. I have watched some who said they were healers approach a person in distress as though they knew where the problem lay. It soon became clear they did not know and that the hand movements were copied from others who may or may not have known better. The healing approach is not to do or say anything that fails to meet the test of reason. And reason is the simple choosing between one course of action or one opinion in preference to another. If you wish to be logical you can trace the mental and emotional steps you took to reach such a choosing. There you may discover whether you used logic, reason, knowledge—or instinct. Healing is not based upon hunches.

Laying on hands has a proper, proved function which is stated in the course of this discussion. It is not to be dismissed without careful thought. What, then, remains is valuable knowledge.

One demonstrated instance of healing at a distance proves that laying on hands is not the only method of applying healing energy to an area of the body, let alone to mental sickness. Since the human mind is known to us only through the brain's physical dimensions and physical substance no one can think of a mind being "handled" as in the laying on of hands. Since the mind is not physical it is more easily reached by spiritual means, that is, by spirit energies at the spirit level of consciousness. Which is a further reason for examining the case for laying on hands according to modern experience.

The role of laying on hands follows after these reflections:

Modern healing by spirits through the agency of mediums trained for the purpose is not new. Some instances of absent healing are reported, for example, in the Bible, but until the recent historical period there is nothing to match the scale of spirit healing of this period.

That era (which is part of this period) is the first in which what are called the occult arts are employed on a wide, public scale for their original purpose: to teach man something of the powers he has, dormant but capable of development. The peculiar and superstitious notions of the occult arts, exploited by churches and priests, have no place in the knowledge of man's inner nature. It is only by demonstrating the benign and healing use of the occult arts, as they are called, that man has begun to discover himself. Psychology, in the best sense, is another approach.

The term "occult" is used because, while the effects of action are known, the causes are veiled from us. The causes are all towards healing; they must be intelligently directed, else there would be no healing art but chaos and chance without prospect of rational assessment.

Modern spirit healing is the only known therapy based upon the occult arts; the power used is transmitted through those who have attuned themselves to become co-operative with spirit intelligences of superior knowledge in controlling and directing the energies used in the art of healing, defined and particular to the need.

Such a declaration will, of course, cause the sophisticated to smile and scoff, because their healing arts depend upon scientific, physical control, repetition and prediction. They seek to engineer for desired results; the healers in the spirit are also scientists, chemists and physicists, as well as physicians. They depend upon human cooperators to provide certain conditions for making contacts with the sick. First of these conditions is a passive awareness. Exercise of will alone, expression of desire, yearning to succeed all inhibit spirit healing and, if continued, lead to failure.

It is easy to understand why such a position arouses resistance since most of us have a touching faith in our ability to control our minds and emotions. Also, there is the lurking fear that we are in some danger by becoming passive. We should study the fruits of the opposite course of life to realise how much wrong has been done by those who live by action alone. We have but to reflect what hurt we do ourselves by our tensions. We have only to reflect on the drug industries developed from the sale of tranquilisers and alcohol to illustrate the errors of "on the go" as a rule of life. We see its effects everywhere. Nothing is fast enough, big enough, loud enough, plentiful enough until we are deafened and rendered insensitive to the needs of our spirit nature by our own desires or by desires thrust upon us. There is no prospect that these words will help change the societies we live in within a lifetime, but it is necessary to point out the facts.

Here is a personal illustration of the value of passivity even in a situation of extreme physical danger:

During World War II I was night editor of a London newspaper. During a long air raid on a clear, moonlit evening, with an assistant I went on the roof—which was forbidden—to see what was happening because of reports of fires. The Germans, at that time, were dropping bombs in clusters of five. We both heard and saw the first four explosions of one group of bombs as they came nearer, when I cried, "Look out, one is coming at us". As we ran we both heard distinct tapping on our steel hats. The last thing we remembered was trying to open the heavy metal door to the elevator head. Nothing else. No more bombs fell, so we went down to the deserted editorial room. Chaos. The bomb we did not hear had sliced through the side of a huge roll of newsprint, pierced the roof and exploded in the editorial room which was a mass of rubble. Force of the explosion switched on the lights. From the street below air raid wardens shouted to us. They were surprised to see we were not hurt. Some short time later I was at a seance with the well known spirit guide, Silver Birch. He mentioned the incident, which I had not told to anyone but my wife. He said: "Next time you are in danger, be still. You make it more difficult for us to help when you run about."

If such an attitude or philosophy prevailed we would have a revolution beyond all other revolutions—without killing or taking advantage of anyone. Imagine, the revolution of the Gentle People! What, then, will we do with our weapons of war and our worship of physical force?

Since all schools of thought begin with contemplation Edwards recommends that healing aspirants shall begin their apprenticeship in contemplation by being seated comfortably upright in a chair with arms, in a dimly lit room when the day's activities are over.

As the radio impulse is carried by a "wave" we should allow our thoughts to be carried on the waves of stillness. As before noted, concentration inhibits healing. Let the mind go, is the guiding rule. We all know how the mind moves from thought to thought until we find we are far from our starting place. The mind will move whether we wish or will otherwise. Our effortless effort is to direct the mind toward contact with spirit people for the purpose of healing. This is the modern, healing application of the urgings of most religions—that we pray constantly.

We are now sitting in a chair that does not cause us to move. Our limbs are also at rest. We will find that our breathing slows down since we do not require the heart to sustain body movement. A few deep breaths will enable us to inhale whatever energy is available. just as we tend to breathe deeply when we are close to nature.

Those who believe they can deliberately attract certain spirit entities by "calling them up" are mistaken —and mislead themselves and others by their demonstrations intended to carry such conviction. We have already much evidence that, given the willing instruments, spirit people will co-operate to effect healing—and other services. My experience is that when the circumstances are appropriate these entities who desire to work with us will make themselves known, even as we become aware. Our prayers, or attuning, will show clearly our state of consciousness. We cannot "make" spirit people come to us. All we can do is to provide the still waters beside which they walk toward us bringing their peace to increase ours. In such harmony we then may address ourselves to our desire to serve. We cannot know how much or little our aspiring to be of service will succeed but we will know, in time, by the effects that manifest in ourselves. We will learn from increasing awareness of spirit influence, from increasing detachment from cares that previously caused us to fear the outcome of our efforts.

Those in the spirit realm I have learned to trust without reservation say that all prayers, all pleas, are known by those closest to us. We humans argue about results as though healing and inspiration were a kind of contest. Sometimes, it is taught, we learn most from the silent answers to our prayers. The silences teach. Where there is a request for healing, it will be answered, not always directly in a spirit message to us, but as the power required is transmitted through the healer.

Edwards, from his lifetime of experience, distinguishes between the objectives of contemplation. Those who desire to heal know the reason for such desire. Where we are motivated by a genuine urge to serve others, with reasonable self-discipline we will achieve good; the measure of good depends upon our potential being realised. In time we will know whether our self-estimate is wise. As we become more attuned to our goals we will become aware of what is to be done, such as perceiving an image or likeness of the person for whom healing is sought.

There are no prizes to be won by skill in contemplation; it is an exercise in relaxation so that whatever power can be made manifest through us will flow with a minimum of resistance.

It is the power that flows to heal, not our thoughts. In time we will know how to direct healing power. We are channels, living channels; instruments, not physical objects; in a sense, one tide flowing within another as do the tides of this world's oceans, an established phenomenon. It is a wonder that so much life can be so diverse, that one aspect is acting as a method of flow while another is the power as it flows. We could well meditate on that wonder as we learn to attune ourselves for more and greater service.

Here is how Edwards explains a healing meditation. It is from his book, *A Guide To Spirit Healing*:

"You are sitting for meditation and for your mind to attune with spirit rather than the attracting of spirit entities to you."

As we pray, or invite spirit presence, we either utter the words in simple form as we are moved, or express ourselves in silent thought.

We should ask for help from the spirit to remove all discord of the body, or spirit, express confidence that good will follow. Guidance and confidence will develop from our sincere approach since these are the natural consequence of our unselfish approach: we attract what we desire most to become—always.

In our contemplation we should conduct ourselves as though we were talking with someone who is listening, always moving in thought outward to the spirit, ourselves open and ready to receive.

Then we should request the listening spirits to remove whatever pain, stress, or illness is affecting the patient. To begin with, each healing approach should be brief, followed by a relaxing period, and, if it appeals, the aspirant may desire to sing softly or hum, keeping in rhythm while envisaging some peace inducing scene such as flowing waters bordered by flowers and trees and the scent which mark such visions, even in the flesh.

As Edwards writes: "And by so doing naturally encourage the spiritual aspect of your nature by thoughts that possess grace and beauty and virtue."

That state he describes as day-dreaming which should develop during contemplation towards spirit healing.

Other guidance in the art of contemplation is given:

"There is no set time as to how long a sitting should continue. At first the minutes will seem to be long, but as the sittings continue the time so spent will be a real pleasure and quickly go, and will be joyfully anticipated during the day. It is further suggested that you do not discipline yourself by fixing a definite time to start the sittings. Let them take place after the daily tasks are comfortably finished. Do not hurry them, but rather see happiness in their accomplishment. Then when you feel the desire to sit for communion with the spirit people, that is the time to do it."

That counsel is, as you will recall, for the guidance of the individual aspirant, not for groups for which it might generate problems, such as time keeping. For myself I find such guidance parallels my own. I find many opportunities to "day dream" and always have done so in the midst of an active life without having been so instructed. It seems that when the daily and required tasks are done the mind can let go its hold upon the consciousness and we can drift, as does a ship tethered to the river bank as the flow of water may dictate. Such is the wonder of the spiritual nature of man that, left to the promptings of the spirit, he will naturally gravitate thence for there is his true home; the tether to the river bank of physical life is a necessary restraint upon the almost impetuous nature of the spirit which always tends towards its home since that is where it dwells in eternity. Such guides as are now given have been known in all times and are brought again to mankind's attention since the condition of contemplation is one of the methods intended for the helping of mankind in its slow and inevitable rising from the deepest physicality to the upward-moving arc of development towards spirituality.

Healing as known on earth is one of the principal modes for educating and regenerating mankind and will one day become a universal. The healing is to repair what has been damaged; once set mankind upon its intended and proper course, free from that condition in which disease, in man and society, abounds, and we may anticipate man in a nobler setting; no longer chained to the rocks of his own hatred but freed, no slave of error and wrongdoing, but a liberated soul dwelling closer to the contemplative life since he will have so reshaped his world that it will begin to resemble that realm to which he tends implacably, free from the need to return to the planet earth, its lessons having been learned, debts paid and the account of evolution balanced, good from evil wrought; wisdom from error fashioned and the spirit, aware and knowing, graduated for further service and joy in the doing of it.

Where a group meets for development, set times will be followed for mutual convenience. For the individual all times where the aspirant is undisturbed and the mind is relaxed are suitable since the spirit co-operators themselves are not bound by time as we are. They are always ready to serve.

Day by day, says Edwards, as we learn to live by the spirit we will learn to "live by a code of true values. You will not do harm to anyone, you will always seek to serve. You will be tolerant in all things and will not allow temper or ill-will to follow any act that may not please you. As you place any displeasing act in its true perspective to life, its relative unimportance will be seen and that it is not worth causing disharmony of mind.

"Help your neighbours by any act of kindness, especially those who are sick and need a word of comfort or an errand undertaken. If during the day you see a sufferer, hold that person in your mind, and then, later, in the quietness, you will ask for help for him."

The healer cites as an example the effect of such an outlook: In an experiment with a friend they sought absent healing for a man suffering from galloping consumption, haemorrhage and pleurisy. He was surprised on learning that within 24 hours bleeding ceased, the pleuritic conditions disappeared, temperature was down to normal; complete cure quickly followed.

Edwards states these principles upon which absent healing is based:

> While you cannot promise yourself (or patients) that any healing result will be seen, it may be that even from the earliest days of your intercession you will observe that sufferers are getting well far more quickly than might have been expected. As this becomes evident so will your healing work have begun.
>
> Speed in establishing spirit communication varies.
>
> No time limit can be set for development; each aspirant is different.

Development is continuous, even with the best mediums.

Attunement long continued becomes second nature —as easy as talking with a friend.

If the aspirant knows of the spirit guide closest to him, his thoughts will naturally go toward him as contemplation begins.

When attunement is achieved the healer will direct the healing through him as freely and naturally as if the sitter were "talking to him by thought".

There is no need to be concerned as to the identities of spirit guides; assurance that "someone" is there should be confirmation that these thoughts are received. He declares: "Hold this knowledge with supreme confidence that it is so. It is quite straightforward, for as you are using your spirit mind so the spirit guides can and do listen in."

Edwards continues with what I regard as the wisest, simplest guidance for potential healers:

"You will not be sitting unless you have the desire to heal. That of itself is a product of your spirit mind. It is a spiritual desire. Therefore, as you sit for this purpose, you can have the fullest confidence that you will be able to tune in with the spirit and that your spirit mentors are waiting for you to do so. It may well be that they have prompted you with the desire to heal and that they are already in touch with you." Counsel on the first stage of healer development ends:

"This, then, is your mental preparation to establish attunement and the first steps in your development as a healer. Do not be in a hurry—a slow development is stronger than a quick growth. The time spent will never be regretted. It will give a serenity of mind and happiness within. As the healing gift is developed and you become an instrument of the spirit to heal the sick, it will be a reward that cannot be measured in material terms."

There is no question that the advent of absent healing is the psychic and spiritual event of the 20th century. The wonder of psychic healing had been known in the Anglo-American community for more than a century through the Spiritualist movement and much earlier in other, smaller groups. But the initiation of absent healing, first through Parish and at one point currently through Edwards brought in a new age of healing, the effects of which are now more widely being recognised.

No intimation was given by the spirit guides of the approaching healing revolution. Whether this was part of a designed approach is not known but if experience in other aspects of Spiritualism are a guide, nothing is done without plan, purpose and the means of achievement.

Cures and betterment resulting from psychic healing by person to person contact were impressive. But when reports of healing at a distance began to be reported, almost wholly in *Psychic News* and other Spiritualist media, the way was opened for what must be described as a revolution; it was a complete turn from the past.

Since Edwards is the most successful healer of the new development, his experience commands the attention of all who would try to follow his example, or study the phenomenon that is changing a large part of world opinion, through media that only a few years ago would have either ignored the cures or would have dealt with them as merely another outburst of what is miscalled faith healing.

We have just reviewed the initial stages of developing healers. Just as the healers in the spirit make contact with those who desire to heal, I believe that long before anyone is moved to desire to heal they are selected to be offered an opportunity to do so. This is true not only of healing but also of other forms of mediumship. The indications of being selected would appear to be shown in the potential medium's gifts. The reverse is true. The gifts, unless close to the surface of consciousness, are stimulated, just as healing forces are mind-directed towards healing. The stirring of spiritual awareness then stimulates the desire to heal, or develop whatever gift or gifts the instrument is to use for a particular service.

In the healer's case it may be stimulated by witnessing a demonstration of healing, by a relative or friend having been healed, or by any of several probabilities. As the aspirant progresses through the stages of contact healing there comes awareness of a further development. Contact healing, already described in its public demonstrations, with all its wonders, deals with the few as compared with the many treated by the absent or distant method.

You are already aware of my lack of enthusiasm for the word "intercession". For me it is a picture of someone pleading for interference with a process deemed harsh; as though someone had broken a religious or civil law. It is true that many diseases arise from breaches of natural law. Even so, the price is paid in pain and other distress. I hold that if we regard the request for absent healing as just that, or as seeking direction of a healing energy, we escape the concept of a suppliant on his knees, or of a plea to a personal deity. I know it will not make any difference to the healing but prefer you know my positions even where they may not be valid.

So, having established a viewpoint . . .

We have already also established the fact that just as modern eminent philosophers in the scientific world admit they are left with thought as the final resource, so, in healing we rely upon thought as the carrier wave of the healing energies. That must be so, since in absent healing most success is achieved when the patient sleeps or when he is unaware of when the healing request through the medium to the healer in spirit is made. Those who challenge these claims cannot maintain their positions in view of the overwhelming evidence.

The medium, in the case of Edwards and previously Parish, does not know precisely what occurs when healing is achieved at a distance. You will recall the American soldier's experience when he was healed by Edwards, then at a distance, in the night. But the healer still does not know what energy was used nor how it was applied. In that instance the healing request was made by a third party for the injured soldier. How did Edwards, in his out of the body experience, know where to go and what to do? Were invisible healers directing him?

I discussed this kind of situation with Parish but made no headway. If one more sleep experience is germane here it is, as an illustration.

I had been thinking of the little I know of the spirit world plan for aiding mankind when, in sleep, I was taken on a journey by someone who propelled me from behind. His face was hidden from me but he took me to a vast area—with white-robed figures, all with their backs to me. Even so, there was an air of intense attention to what they were doing. The groups, widely separated, I was told, were all engaged in a spirit plan to influence progressive minds on earth. With the assurance that I need not worry about what was being done was well done, the scene changed and I was informed that many on earth are aware of such influences; that groups each have their tasks and that we should all "get on with it". I did not see one face, nor hear a sound, had no sense of location, and to this day can recall the entire experience. I imagine many have such experiences which, in substance, are not different from the Parish and Edwards excursions on their healing missions. And still the healing process itself is not disclosed.

Here in substance is what occurs:

> Applications for healing come by letter, telephone or in person either from the person involved or someone concerned for him or her.
>
> The healer responds during his quiet period for absent healing, alone or with associates.
>
> According to his development or natural gifts the required state of attunement is achieved.
>
> The healer's full confidence that his mental request to his spirit guides on behalf of the patient will be received is essential.
>
> Although by nature most of us have the absent healing gift, realised or potential, the successful healer/medium has prepared himself for his work through the development of his psychic gifts by living as closely as he may according to spiritual values.
>
> Since confidence begets competence, as we associate closely with the spirit intelligence, so does the ease and fullness of communication come into play.

It was not until this part was reached that it occurred to me the experience with the medium, John Myers, was an instance of a thought appeal for healing registered with a spirit guide and that he influenced Myers to change direction and come to my home. Only now, after many years, do I realise that the guide heard or somehow knew and was aware of my wife's predicament and came ready to direct the healing which shows that Edwards' claim has evidence other than his own and that we who have so much experience have evidence heaped and overwhelming before we even know its force and meaning. If this were not so, why were we given the preliminary notice on the piece of photographic paper: "Watch for Good Friday", some days in advance of the healing?

The question of thought communication is proved over and over. Still the world of science and medicine is little moved; they require a machine to prove a truth when the most remarkable instrument ever devised for man is man himself.

Edwards maintains that contact between spirit guide and patient may be the least of his problems. The healer's spirit self can travel swifter than light to the patient; so can the spirit doctor's. The healer in spirit must make contact more easily since he does not have to allow for the medium's peculiarities. The guides operate in their own environment while they contact a patient at the request of the healer/medium.

Another situation now develops: The ability of the healing guide to deal with the patient where the physical and spirit bodies are out of harmony. This discord shows up in either the mind or the body. It is one of the spirit guide's functions in absent healing to diagnose, or he cannot heal. Once diagnosis is done the process of restoring harmony begins; then the body and mind are in a sounder relationship, and healing is on its way.

Patients may have either physical problems, such as broken bones, burns, infections, or other injuries, or maybe a problem of spirit imbalance, or a combination of both. It is easy to see which problems arise in the spirit nature. It could be that the healing spirits administer their equivalent of medication once the discords are removed and harmony begins. Removal of tumours is not difficult to visualise since we are convinced that "occult" energy is successfully applied by spirits to situations with which surgeons cannot deal save by their earthbound conditions. Here is a new, large and intricate field of research.

I know of an instance of a brain tumour being removed or dissolved by spirit healing. Others have evidence of such cures. In the one known to me, again the medium was John Myers, certainly not a brain surgeon. The patient's tumour was medically diagnosed. He was employed in the Buckingham Palace maintenance unit.

Myers had remarkable cures of many others. So far as I am aware—and we were close friends—he did not, at any time, undergo any particular self-discipline or careful study. No men could be more different than Jones, Myers, Parish and Edwards. Each is unique. Each demonstrated the superb gifts they came with; each has a place in the invisible hall of fame built of service to others even when they are not recognised either by their time or in the unwritten history of Spiritualism. Each has a share in changing thought by serving as an instrument of the spirit by healing mind and body; in bringing the great news of Survival beyond death; in being an agent for the cure of many diseases, and in ending fear of death.

The purpose of that evaluation is to show that there is a spirit power in this world, at work, now and forever, varied according to the changes in people and in society, in nations and in groups of nations. That Edwards is the latest and most successful is, in part, due to the efforts of all who beat the path he has followed and to tread extensions of that path for the armies of healers who are to come.

And when our generation has served its season brief upon this earth we will, as was done with us, stay our forward passage, as others have stayed their progress for us in order that the oncoming souls may live closer to the spirit, better, nobler, more kind, more humane, less cruel, more tolerant than we could achieve because our times were harder.

I am not in a position nor of a mind to settle nicely an order of ranking among such men. As Isaac Newton said when honoured by his peers for his achievements, "I but stood on the shoulders of giants". We, who are largely anonymous but also serve silently, are privileged to live so long in the company of those who were by the spirit raised up to stand on the shoulders of such spiritual giants as that band of disciples who gave their lives in following one who was not permitted to do more than change history before his spirit was thrust untimely from his body.

I am compelled to pause in this narrative to make a point: that the power of the spirit rules; that there is not now and nevermore shall be any authority vested in any woman or man, or in any aggregation of women and men, that will control the coming, upraising and expression of spirit power. The men so far named are an earnest of that truth: each is unique; the service they rendered is the same: to heal the sick and comfort the mourner. That is all. It is everything that is asked of them.

To resume the story: It now is clear that the body, the psychic nature and the spirit (or soul) interact one upon the other in a resonance, or sounding of cause-effect; effect-cause and in such harmony as may be achieved in all the abrasions and consolations of this life upon earth. The environment in which that holy trinity lives is thought. In its evolution thought, the expression of mind, has broken down barriers of ignorance and superstitition. It is not enough to strike down such barriers; thought, organised and left to run free, must be shaped by our souls so that we move closer to the spirit of life. Many systems have been devised to express these concepts, none endures since thought's vehicle of expression is change and the laws of change are themselves always on the move towards greater expression: to the goal that one day, the race of women and men will be as they all dream in their secret hearts. Such is the opportunity offered all when they come to consider; What is the use of teaching there is no death, and, what is the use of healing if I am well?

Among the distilled advice given by Edwards is that healers should think with purpose, that is, never allot the casual to replace the deliberately invoked healing power. This casualness, he stresses, is greatest when healers seek aid for themselves on the assumption that close association with the spirit guides enables them to acquire what may be called the "house spirit guide" as some have their own "house doctors". The same caution is given against the casual expectation of "healing on tap" for members of the healer's family, as though the guides are hanging around waiting for something to happen that may require their service—unsought. Edwards' summation is: Where casualness rules healing seldom occurs.

All of the foregoing is to emphasise the fundamental nature of the metaphysical. Healers in the spirit use thought to effect changes in consciousness—which we call healing. It could be that we have been dwelling on energy and force when it could be that the "secret" healing power is thought itself. Is not "thought" also "energy and force"? Earlier on it was mentioned that a Japanese researcher had photographed a medium's thoughts. Perhaps I am too hasty in reaching opinions. Maybe the photographs show only the effect of thought since to see thought itself is beyond human perception.

It is clear that the resource of healing is in thought, as the source of all human action is thought, whether it be in movement of the limbs, of the internal functions of the body, or of the activity of the brain. When the time in evolution is ripe we will, through the mind, comprehend thought as we cannot understand it now; the mind, I believe, is, like all other aspects of consciousness, moving towards self-recognition or self-consciousness.

**Since healing is built on thought it is idle to conduct rituals or make gestures as priests, and some healers do, to induce change. Thought obeys laws; rituals do not affect laws.**

Just as the casual approach to healing is self-inhibiting, so does the structured approach inhibit; that is the practice of setting times when patients should seek to link their thoughts with the healer/medium's. The lesson learned from such procedures, as Edwards discovered, is that they induce tension based upon expectation—natural but not helpful.

It is the aim that both healer and recipient should be as passive as possible when help is sought since the guides depend upon our state of consciousness and not upon the clock. As a practical matter it is unwise to expect a patient to develop skill in passivity when his need is, at most, occasional whereas the healer/medium seeks to attain his goal through years of preparation. It is as though a beginner on the violin should be expected to give a concert after the first few lessons. Therefore, where the appeal for healing has been made, the patient should relax since he cannot know when he is being treated. His request is registered through the healer; the guides carry out their duty according to their time and their way of serving. Pain, clocks and domestic arrangements interfere with the emergence of the passive condition—best in sleep, best achieved when we live as the world lives.

Edwards has the best experience for giving such guidance in the matter of passivity. Here is a summary of his procedure as followed by himself and his personal assistant healers, Mr. and Mrs. George Burton, who have co-operated with him for 27 years.

No time appointments are made.

The healer makes requests early in the morning or late at night after the day's activities are over. Healing requests continue until all are dealt with.

Direct requests are made, mentally, for each of the known disharmonies, or conditions; some conditions are stated by patients in their required weekly reports;

in addition spirit knowledge is given. Healing continues while weekly reports are made, except where application is made from abroad, for third parties living at a distance, or where a patient is in an institution.

All requests for healing are answered.

Where healing is directed to a specific condition the more effective is the healing.

The healer registers requests. These give rise to mind pictures of the patient, even of his physical location, his condition; then the subconscious is primed to make the information available to the spirit guides. It is not difficult to imagine a "behind the scenes" picture of the process.

The newcomer will ask: If the spirit guides do what is claimed and exhibit superior knowledge and power, why do they require such a procedure as outlined above? Edwards replies: ". . . healing most often takes place in the spirit self of the patient". As the spirit guide or physician operates at that level he may not always be aware of what is happening in the physical body.

I have been told by Silver Birch, known widely and with affection, that he used the power available to him for communication alone. He does not see us physically, he says, but he sees our spirit bodies and from their appearances learns how we respond to his statements. He hears and speaks. He does not see us physically. It is a lesson of economy in the use of energy. He does know, from frequent control of his medium's body, what is its condition. By the way, his medium, Maurice Barbarell, has not had a day's illness in more than 40 years as a trance medium. Edwards has never had a day's illness and has never needed the services of a doctor.

During the healer's statement of patients' conditions the spirit healers often provide diagnoses which are "invariably correct".

To understand more clearly the need for the healer/medium to provide pertinent data for the healer/guides consider: patients come and go. Their cases are given the healing available and relevant. Most patients are either cured or experience improvement. Then, even where healing is continued for a time, they are no longer included in the healer's daily request sessions. But, in the case of the trance medium/healer the relationship with the guide is often so close that reports are not required. The healer/medium's role is that of the doctor of first instance: to provide essential data for a specialist. And in the spirit there are many specialists.

We have already covered the psychic gift Edwards uses to travel outside the body to gather information on patients seeking healing and on his ability to "photograph" conditions and to recall every detail without concentration. This phenomenon shows how the mind, which is a spirit organ, extends its capacity to effect healing, once the healer achieves the necessary inner tranquillity. The spirit mind is attracted to the patient—only for the purposes of healing. Whether spirit guides are involved in the exercise of this gift of out of the body travel, I do not know.

Those who aspire to become healers should study the literature on the subject. Many books are written that could profit them. Only those gifted, trained, tried by experience and with records of success beyond doubt should be heeded. No one would hire a lawyer known to be ignorant of the law, nor engage a surgeon or a bricklayer or a carpenter unless satisfied that each knew his trade. It is a peculiarity of those who write books on subjects miscalled metaphysical, divine healing or the like, seldom speak from direct, personal, verifiable experience.

My voice is small but whenever it can be raised I call in question the qualifications of those who without regard to consequences set up as mediums and healers. It is true that in return for freedom of expression we must be ready to put up with much mediocrity. Yet, even many who are highly regarded as authorities are merely providers at third or tenth hand of unverified information. The willingness of many of us to believe without evidence is shown in the gross errors of many who have written about healing without knowledge. Some defend their actions by pointing out that doctors also make mistakes, that is true—and universal. But mistakes may be corrected by increased experience. What hurts is that deliberate ignorance is sold as a remedy when knowledge is available. I have seen so much that thrives upon credulity that I could wish for some method of correction.

Elsewhere Edwards states the case this way: When anyone makes it known that he or she is a healer, that claim will attract sufferers. When the healer does heal, he will be occupied healing. When his claim to heal falls short, the diseased will go elsewhere.

The foregoing is prelude to adding that in addition to studying the literature on healing, the inquirer should make his study comprehensive and choose which method he will follow, if that is his intent. Fortunately, all healers are not authors, else I might try to become a healer.

Information is available to guide you if you desire to heal. To my mind the best instructional material available today is written by Edwards because he has most experience plus a gift of clear explanation. If I knew of a better teacher, this would be a book about him. Since Edwards is an unassuming man, he will understand this is a sincere attempt to foster healing at the highest level in this period of development.

Edwards, in his early work, published *A Guide To Spirit Healing*. My copy is from the 13th impression

(1969). That guide is the best book I know of on healing as a service to mankind. I recommend its study. It is not offered as a gospel or as a bible: it is a guide based upon the experience of one who has not only given his life to it but has asked all the questions necessary to ensure that he has the answers fitting the facts as far as they have been discovered. It has been revised and enlarged to include knowledge of greater experience and is now titled *A Guide to the Understanding and Practice of Spiritual Healing*.*

I cannot reproduce all of Edwards' statements. His guide is detailed. We move as speedily now to present the points that appeal to me and stated as I understand them:

Among the questions asked of me is this one: Since so much is said about absent healing why use contact healing?

The answer is that, because the human hand is, by instinct, the first contact we make with one another. The hand can be many things. It is without superior as a physical transmitter of healing power at the physical level and as a sensor of the patient's health. Mothers soothe their children by a caress—or check them with the opposite. We greet one another by hand. You can finish the list for yourself; it will be instructive. The healing hand is a fact, in the sense that it is superbly sensitive. As Edwards sets out his guidance you will learn why he writes so carefully about "healing passes" and "wiping away" disease. He examines his own views —which are not the accepted views. Indeed, Edwards has always been a pioneer, to me, since he cleared my mind on the doubts I had about "faith healing". I remember that incident as clearly as the words I now write.

* Published by the Healer Publishing Co. Ltd., Burrows Lea, Shere, Surrey. £2.75 post inc.

He deals with the claim that health conditions are shown in the human aura, and that there is a method of "cleansing" the aura.

I have tried some of the things he deals with and in doing so felt embarrassed. That was because I was repeating the errors of others and had not inquired as to the facts. Also, the results did not match expectations. Many of us err when we say the hands heal; only the spirit heals; hands are channels of spirit healing.

**Remove the spirit power and the hands are hands.**

Then there is the hoary theory that passes are made to throw off disease—as though it were a thing. If you study the Edwards book you will understand why he is emphatic on his experience.

"The sole use of hand movements," he writes, "is that they are expressive of the mental desire of the healer to erase the pain and to this extent they may be useful."

I have been in trouble, when teaching, by saying that the upward gaze, the upturned palms and so on have nothing to do with healing while closing the eyes helps relaxation and that energy will flow as easily from the back of the hand as the palms.

Finally on making passes: "Thus it is seen that the actual healing value of passes is discounted. No physical movement, as such, can produce the healing results."

Remember, there are no hand passes in absent healing. That should make us think. My own view is that the healer/medium is the alternative to the direct application of spirit power which is more direct when the passive condition is complete. Even the most co-operative medium cannot be 100 per cent passive.

But, and here is a seeming anomaly: In a further phase

of the healer's development it is stated there is no single method whereby skill in diagnosis may be achieved. Some healers, it appears, receive an image of the body area requiring attention; the disharmony itself may be "seen", or a picture of a heart situation appears. Diagnosis and healing follow. Some healers see a radiance or a light over the part requiring attention. Where the healer is entranced the spirit guide can provide diagnosis and treatment.

Other diagnostic methods are by light touch over the patient's body (contact is not essential) so that a sensation may be felt; it is either warm or cold, indicating a transfer of energy. Where the sensation is strongest, that is the trouble area. Thermometers do not register these temperature changes (as you may recall in the Mr. E case when tested by closely controlled scientific methods).

"Angry" conditions, perhaps inflammations, usually exude heat but this is not to be confused with the healing heat found during diagnosis. Heat intensity decreases with distance of the hand from the affected area; this heat is clearly non-physical, a condition not denied in science.

Edwards says that intuitive diagnosis frequently is the best way to locate the cause of disease and that as the beginner gathers experience his mind becomes more receptive and information is more readily provided. Medical or other terms for the diseases are given in time, not always in the orthodox classifications but sufficient; only the healing matters, not the terms. In time the healer will be able to discuss the diagnosis with the patient.

These are bare outlines to be supported by experience. There is, apparently, no limit to the development of a healer: he or she never need fear "running out" of the need to make progress.

But, there is this comfort; it is always a question for the

beginner whether to continue when the phenomena of success do not manifest. We all seek for a sign. A small happening buoys up our expectations which if long deferred frequently lead to loss of interest. In the case of the developing healer he should find some encouragement in knowing that his progress is increasing, little by little, and that he has the incentive of knowing that in his quiet times he is achieving the goal—the beginning of attunement, much to be yearned for, apart from its imperative need as a basis for healing. Each small step brings the aspirant closer to his first healing.

What are the causes of disease? There are many theories and some facts. Since we have, together I hope, seen that the mind is the soul's prime mover, we should be aware of the perfect response of the psychic and physical natures to the mind's action. This happening is recognised in the belief of most thoughtful physicians that the mind-body interaction (psychomatic) is at the root of causes of disease. We daily experience stress, anger, fear and the other emotions. Spirit healing has achieved a major breakthrough by demonstrating the reality of the mind—and science is silent—science which has no resource beyond thought.

What kind of a world could we have if science and the spiritual were in unity? This is not a distant dream. The British Medical Association does not yet acknowledge spirit healing; it mildly supports church healing. An increasing number of physicians support spirit healing and send their patients to healers. Hospitals send patients to Edwards. Healers desire liaison and co-operation with doctors. One day the conservative BMA will be impelled to join in with spirit healers, for no truth can be buried for ever.

We have made inroads into the territory formerly ruled by orthodoxy. The opportunity is here. The knowledge is available, the case is proved, the need is demonstrated.

What are we waiting for? Only for the steady increase in the number of healers.

The triumph of spirit healing is well worth the years of toil. We did not and do not labour alone. The vast, silent army of the Gentle People in the spirit world is with us. Who, then, can prevail against us?

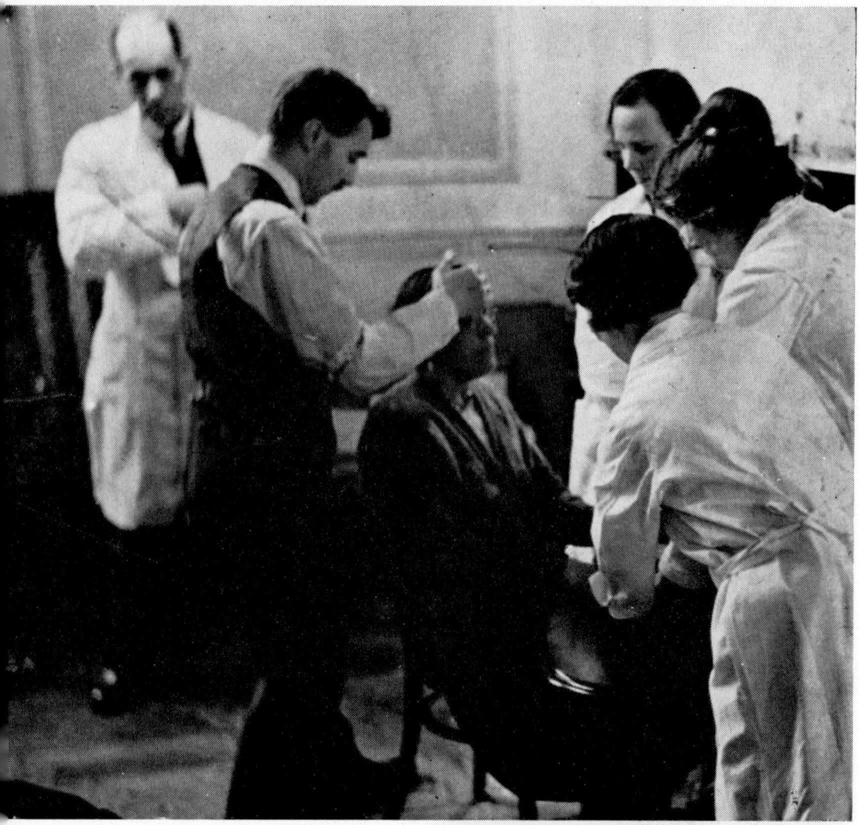

FRED J. JONES

Pioneer of modern healing and medium of 'Medicine Man'. He worked while in trance, treating up to 400 patients daily, each one by personal contact. Above picture is of Jones healing in his sanctuary.

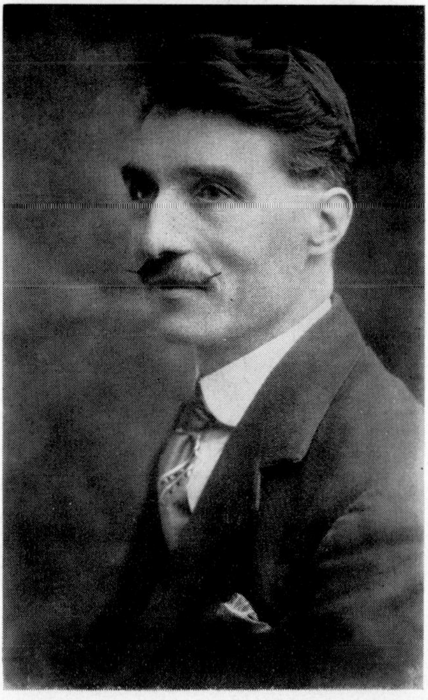

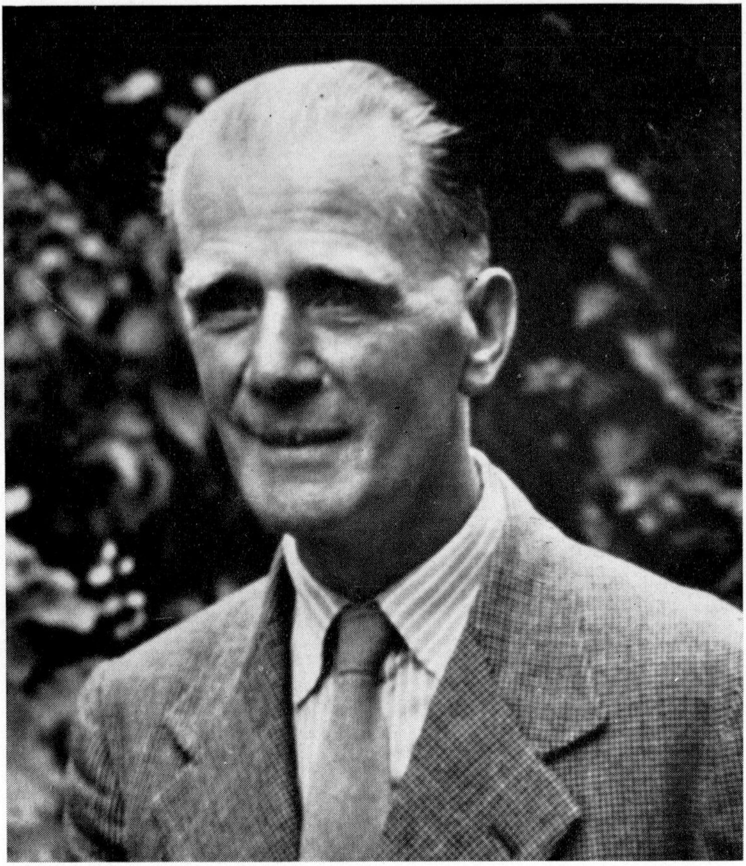

BILLY PARISH

One of the trinity of great spirit healers of our time. He became a healer after curing his wife of cancer. A pioneer in absent, or distant, healing.

THE THREE MODERN
PIONEERS OF
SPIRIT HEALING

FRED JONES
BILLY PARISH
HARRY EDWARDS

## JONES, FIRST OF MODERN HEALING MOVEMENT

The three healers selected as signposts of progress in the unfolding mission of spiritual healing through mediums are representative and not exclusive. Many others could be added to the three—Jones, Parish and Edwards—but, since there must be limits, I thought it wiser to tell the story of those who touched most people. There is no order of ranking in what follows.

In the early days of my interest in spirit healing there was no awareness of the long-range purpose upon which healing was developed. It was known that healing had been a spirit-inspired service as long as man had learned the art of living so as to develop disease. No disease, no healing. Healing is a service to remedy the defects in man and in his societies. It is partly therapeutic but mostly a form of education based upon demonstrated revelation.

I say revelation since no one could have arrived at the scientific aspects by logical means alone. As in other areas of human development, all reform or discovery must begin with an idea arising from a human need. No one could have thought out spirit healing as we now know it: the knowledge arose from the necessity, the imperative need to change from the undesirable state called disease to the desirable state called health.

All disease is a form of malfunction brought on by breach of spiritual and natural laws. From that premise it is a simple task to understand what are called the mysteries of heredity; at some point in the evolution of a soul a law or laws were broken. The iron laws of consequence were then set in motion and we learned to live, more or less agreeably, with the disease condition. Whether the laws are breached knowingly or not, the consequences follow.

Disease is a warning that something is in breach of laws, spiritual and natural. From such a primal statement events and consequences follow until we observe a rational explanation of what ails us. The rational explanation of revelation as healing is arrived at in a study of the millions of cases of appeals for spirit healing in the past half century alone. That is another reason why only three healers are chosen as signposts: the basic facts are simply stated, the statistics are compelling and the healing itself cannot be explained other than on the terms stated by the healers in the spirit world and supported by demonstrated factual events called healings and evidence of a whole world of thought and remedial service.

In the course of this work it is stressed that spirit healing, that is, healing initiated and directed by discarnate persons, is a progressive development long planned by advanced spirits. The purpose of that healing, which is wider and deeper than curing disease and relieving many kinds of emotional and mental distress, is to change human thought and conduct more nearly to that of our spiritual counterparts.

It is my hope that these aims have been clearly stated. It is also my hope that the evidence presented is, at least, more than sufficient to establish a logical, rational case.

Elsewhere it is stated that, in modern times, in Britain alone, the three signpost healers are Fred J. Jones, W. T. Parish and Harry Edwards. Earliest of the three is Jones, but this is not to say that these three alone are the sum of the spirit healing and teaching mission.

They are the three outstanding healers of our time by reason not only of their curative and ameliorative services but because they demonstrated further evidence of purpose, a question that vexes many who take a merely, or mainly, intellectual position in regard to the vast body of psychic evidence for human survival of death.

A purpose for human experience on this earth is doubted by many, denied by some and deeply pondered by most, especially when we suffer pain. When all goes well there is no stimulus to cause reflection. That is the situation into which all religions have plunged and have emerged with responses that do not answer the continuing WHY? Into that situation the service called spiritual healing was slowly introduced. That story of the origins of modern Spiritualism is amply told elsewhere. The purpose here is to present the case for the nature, origin, development and long-range purpose upon which spiritual healing is offered to mankind and to record some of its effects.

In deciding to deal with the three signpost healers, Jones, Parish and Edwards, the challenging questions of purpose and motive could not be avoided. Since the question of purpose is put, the answer, based upon the evidence, is that it is to advance the development of all mankind by showing that we are now and forever spirits wearing bodies, bodies that in themselves are wonders beyond telling.

Our bodies are marvels, yet the spirit that animates them is more marvellous still.

Then, if the body is sick and cannot serve its controlling spirit, the great WHY question is inevitable. There are many therapies available to man, few that are wholly concerned with his spirit. There is no call here to be diverted to a study of medicine. The materials for such study are available to all. Our purpose is to show that there is another therapy—the power of the spirit which is not under human control and direction but requires human mediumship for its effective use.

By providing, over nearly a century and a half that we do survive death, we are in a position to say that there is no conceivable limit to evolution. The purpose in healing sick minds and bodies is not only to relieve pain but to inspire new concepts to persuade all of us that we are spirits now. Spirit healing is one more service devised by superior beings to teach us how to love, in all respects, so that we may more fully express our spiritual natures.

Since no person can by him or herself generate the spirit power that heals, and since no person can precisely direct the power that heals, then there must be a Something, some advanced intelligence. Somewhere, somehow there must be human spirits beyond the flesh with the knowledge and power to heal and with a scientific knowledge and superb artistry in applying that knowledge.

That Something is revealed in all the phenomena already described, in all of the personal experiences told, and it is made manifest in all the evidence piled high of the wonderful work of spirit healing, by spirits discarnate through spirits incarnate, to benefit other incarnate spirits.

The wonder is that the healing grows and changes the lives of many from despair and pain to a condition of wholeness, calmness and, frequently, to a desire to heal others.

It is also clear that the claim that God will always provide witness to our spiritual nature is founded on certainty since in healing there is proof that it does not depend upon the authority claimed by orthodoxy. The three modern signpost healers, Jones, Parish and Edwards, have made the record and upon their service others will build.

Frederick Joseph Jones was remarkable for his simplicity, his humility and his dedication. His ministry of healing lasted only 11 years. At its peak he healed some 23,000 annually—mostly in person. He is little remembered now except by veteran Spiritualists but he is indeed a spirit healing signpost.

Jones' spirit guide, Medicine Man, a Zulu of powerful personality, has been pictured—and seen clairvoyantly by many. I have the honour of knowing many spirit guides with unusual names much like Medicine Man; all are beings of a superior nature.

Medicine Man stated, during his relatively brief mission, carried out through a man of almost fanatical devotion, that he had for a century prepared himself for his work.

The best account I have found of the Medicine Man–Jones healing comes from a personal record kept at the time by John F. Wheeler, the Brother John of *Psychic News*, whose gentle philosophy has been given, week by week, for more than 20 years.

The healing of Wheeler's mother, which brought him into the Medicine Man healing band, was typical of that entity's astonishing service. Brother John, at the time of his writing, properly says that Jones was a trance medium. He spent several hours each day entranced while Medicine Man did the healing.

At that time, the early thirties, there was little mention of absent healing as we know it now. That came into prominence soon, with the emergence of Billy Parish.

Neither Parish nor Edwards healed in the trance state. That was a marked development.

Since Brother John was one of the band of Jones' group of healers his testimony is valuable, the more so because of the careful records he kept. He is a perceptive witness. His account of Jones' humble origins shows again that, in most cases, the Spiritualist healers originated either in what we call working class, or close to it. My belief is that this is evidence of intent, since the essential early discipline of hardship tends to sweeten the nature of a potential healer and render it more responsive to the need for compassion which is at the heart of healing. Jones admirably expressed these qualities.

For many years Jones earned his living as a builder and decorator. His first direct intimation of the healing was when, as a member of a circle for psychic development he clairaudiently heard a voice asking whether he would consent to become a healing medium. That work he began in a small group in Wimbledon, with six patients.

The spirit who made the original proposal that Jones become a healer gave the American Indian name, Quiverfoot, then showed himself. A neighbour brought his ailing wife to Jones. Her complaint was epilepsy, caused by shock. She had been treated by two doctors for two years without improvement. The spirit, Quiverfoot, treated the woman on one condition; if she agreed to give time to Jones' work she would be cured. She was cured and devoted her life to co-operation in the healing.

This American Indian controlled Jones in his trance healing for two years, explaining that he was working under a more advanced spirit. This was Medicine Man who, at first, did not speak English but as many spirits do, soon learned.

The Jones mission grew until at Marylebone House, headquarters of the Marylebone Spiritualist Association (now the Spiritualist Association of Great Britain), he treated up to 400 sufferers on two days weekly and probably as many again on other days elsewhere.

In the healing band, so frequently a feature in the work of most mediums of that kind, were 16 others trained to co-operate. Some, like the woman healed of epilepsy, had been cured and in turn became healers. Jones did not take fees, receiving only a small portion of the collections made at Marylebone House. He did not take fees at healing meetings elsewhere, although occasionally some grateful patient would insist on his taking a gift. His dedication was the secret of his success. Literally he died young because he did too much considering his physical constitution.

Two episodes stand out amid all the relief he brought to many thousands. One instance is of a doctor, colleague of a well known Harley Street specialist, who sent 12 patients to Jones for diagnosis by Medicine Man. The doctor attended two healing meetings to observe the Zulu diagnose. Ten of the 12 cases were diagnosed correctly, one was said to be wrong. The doctor concerned re-examined that case in light of the spirit diagnosis and concluded it was accurate.

Jones appeared in court once, at Woking, charged under the old Vagrancy Act. A man who had received medical care for his heart trouble over many years consulted Medicine Man. The patient improved so much that he ran a poultry farm. One year later he died of influenza. Since a doctor had not been called, an inquest was held. The verdict was "death from heart failure".

One month later Jones appeared before the Woking magistrates. But they were so impressed by his healing successes, as stated in evidence by many patients, that the case was stopped and the charge dismissed.

Medicine Man said he was supported by a team of doctors, scientists and chemists, and that he had a laboratory for his work. It is easy to understand this would be so in view of the facts already set out concerning information from other spirit healers.

The Zulu healer had his own methods. While the medium was entranced the guide would place a handkerchief on a patient's back and blow through it. Questioned, he said he was applying the breath of life. Here is one detailed account of a Medicine Man "handkerchief healing", from a *Psychic News* article by Frank Hawken, then secretary of the Marylebone Spiritualist Association.

It is the story of Doreen, aged four, who developed meningitis following measles. Her parents were told the child was near death. A specialist confirmed the attending physician's diagnosis. He saw little hope. In despair the parents called for a second opinion; this confirmed the other two medical opinions. The third doctor said: "Just let her lay, keeping her face bathed until the end, for nothing can be done".

The child's grandmother, from whose diary the whole account is summarised, had benefited much from spirit healing, was called in. A relative was sent to Marylebone House to consult Medicine Man. He magnetised a handkerchief by his breathing therapy, telling the child's relative to place it on her immediately, and that if she could sleep through the night it could lead to recovery.

As soon as the handkerchief was placed on the child's face her distress subsided; temperature fell the next day. Another handkerchief treated by Medicine Man was placed on the child the following day. On the day following the family doctor was "mystified" by the child's improvement. He called it "marvellous". He was not told of the spirit healing.

When Jones called on the little patient, the healer was

entranced. Medicine Man said he would draw pus from the child through the back of the head and asked that her hair be shaved. He instructed the parents that when the wounds appeared, they should be treated by a mixture of olive oil and chalk.

That evening pus was discharged from a number of points, as forecast by the guide. Two days later the family doctor called. He did not interfere. He was told the grandmother had applied an African remedy. For days after that, the doctor said it was a miracle the child had survived.

Twice later Jones gave the child contact healing. Her lost speech returned, and one week later was running "all over the place" when she was taken to Marylebone House. The medical statements were full. The record is clear—Doreen was saved by a Zulu healer in the spirit, in co-operation with a dedicated healer in the flesh.

So, Jones, who came from the people, served them with all his gift of healing, and gave them his life in service.

As Jones passed from this earth to rejoin those who sent him, among them, Medicine Man, another man of the people, Billy Parish, was entering the work for which he came. Jones died in 1933 aged 48, leaving his wife and two children. Only the older generation of Spiritualists remember Jones. I discovered that during research in preparing this record so that, at least, the work of the healing pioneers would not be entirely forgotten on earth.

## PARISH

Parish is the second healer in the three chosen for discussion. His emergence is seen to have followed almost immediately on the ending of the Jones mission which had many intriguing aspects. Parish, like Edwards, began with a background directly opposed to the spiritual concepts they later developed as a result of direct, personal experience of their spirit teachers and healers.

Most of us come to the spirit view of life opposed; by revelation and the education of experience we evolve a philosophy meeting all our needs, a philosophy that reconciles the opposite poles of thought and establishes a universal concept in which all contradictions are reconciled, wherever and in whatever manner they exist.

Since the grand aim of the spirit world's plan for mankind is to help us achieve our spiritual regeneration, progress must be slow as we measure time. Centuries become moments in evolution. Hence the missions of Jones, Parish and Edwards have the stamp of their origins in that they demonstrate a basic quality—service without discrimination or exploitation.

The reader will, in going thus far, have developed a series of questions which in one way or another are answered, in part, in these pages. It is better that the reader should shape his questions and challenges for only then can he measure his receptivity or resistance; in either way he will have achieved an opinion different from that in which he began.

The three healers did not begin as children reared in an atmosphere of belief in the spirit world as outlined here; quite the opposite. They, assuming this story is authentic, had each to endure the normal stresses and strains of life at an economic level which barred them from what is called higher education of the kind that qualifies men and women to become professionals.

That being so, how did Parish, for example, rise to eminence as a healer in co-operation with beings in the spirit world? He had become a railroad executive when his wife developed cancer. One breast was removed. During convalescence she noted that each time he visited her she, and other women in a like situation, felt markedly better. None knew why. Mrs. Parish was told that the cancer would recur and that she had only some six months to live.

Parish, known to thousands as Billy, is my close friend, therefore, I must write of him with restraint lest love clouds judgment. He had no interest in Spiritualism—or in healing. His work took him away from home frequently. During one such absence Mrs. Parish was urged by a Spiritualist to seek spirit healing. Billy was opposed: "Spiritualism is only for weak-minded women and for men who don't think" was his response.

The wife won. Together she and Parish visited a Spiritualist church. He, though well-read, had no knowledge of the psychic case—hence his sweeping view. Now he heard something of the facts. They went again to the little church and read Spiritualist literature. He prayed for guidance. It soon came.

The Parish pair, at their first seance with a medium they did not know, received a spirit communication from a "dead" doctor. He spoke of Mrs. Parish's operation, told Billy he was a born healer. It was his initiation into the service of healing. Said the doctor who had passed from earth to the spirit world: "You will be used for the healing of your own wife".

From instructions then given by the spirit, Billy applied himself, reporting progress steadily for nine months. When duties called him from home he treated his wife despite the distance between them. Often, he said, he was aware of the presence of the dead doctor and others whose identities he later established. By absent treatment and laying on hands, Mrs. Parish was cured.

To test the reliability of that claim I had Parish arrange that I interview the specialist who had removed the cancerous breast. I asked him whether he agreed with the claim that spirit healing was the cause of curing the condition in the other breast. He said that was his belief. Would he sign an affidavit to that effect? Yes, he would, therefore, I did not request it. His word was enough.

So, the forecast by the spirit was achieved and the healing mission of William T. Parish began. He had always been athletic so, it is claimed, was almost ideal as a healer. Yet I know of healers who, in some ways, are as effective as Parish was, if not in numbers of cures, who were not athletic. Indeed I know one who almost enjoys lack of exercise yet is hale and busy. The rule seems to be that we do not know all the rules to be followed by healers in their habits except that they should avoid what obviously is unhealthy, including tension and fear of any kind, and that they should be loyal to their colleagues and to the truths they have been given.

It is because I desire to present great healers as fallible men who achieve great deeds through the spirit and not by their own innate knowledge and power that this frank statement is made.

Leaving names aside, for obvious reasons, here is a personal experience. When I lived in London for some 20 years, I contended with agonising migraine headaches, due, I believe, to the pressures of journalistic work. Migraines are a family complaint, so I assumed heredity was the explanation. Of course, there were those who told me it was due to my karma, which is a complex situation that is beyond my knowledge.

In a personal study, while I laboured on a London morning newspaper, the habits of colleagues were noted. They, too, were under like strains. They all drank and smoked too much. They all were meat eaters, took little exercise, did not meditate. Not one had migraine headaches. They broke all the "rules". Why did I have them? To the best of my knowledge I am as free from fear as anyone I have met; death to me is an adventure. Some friends are confident I must be mistaken in my convictions. Some have asked why my spirit friends didn't cure the migraines.

Another view of the conditions required of the healer: I was asked to speak on healing to a church group. A migraine headache developed early that day; the directions to the church were confusing. When the discussion period began several in the small audience said they had been healed; two women thanked me because their migraines had stopped; mine continued till the next day.

Finally the migraine tendency was healed—by my forgetting to be tense.

To achieve a continuing condition of absence of tension is but the beginning of self-healing.

In moving from one conditioning of consciousness to another there cannot be any gaps or vacuums since there is no emptiness in space or matter, therefore, no vacancy in consciousness. The conditioning is all, as it speaks eloquent of movement towards achieving a closer nearness to the more desirable and inevitable states of spirituality.

I believe this since it chimes with my inner experiences arising from an ending to a lifelong war within myself. As the tensions of this world lessened so did the inner peace expand until in silent moments and alone ecstasy rose from the depths. Then the obverse side of the coin of consciousness appeared, bright with gleaming gold; what is pain on one side is ecstasy on the other, and which aspiring soul would not gladly suffer the pain of migraine rampant for the peace and joy triumphant?

I am aware that to many this confession of a faith based upon knowledge will appear a strange thing. Nonetheless, it is so, else I know nothing, have endured nothing and deceive myself as to the joy that springs from peace won at so hard a price that if foretold would cause the aspirant to shrink at his own hardihood and vanity. But as one step begins a great journey upon a spiritual enterprise so do I, in full view of my spirit guides and friends, testify that healing is of the spirit, that it has no bounds and is the spirit's witness to the love that will not be denied and is mankind's greatest hope.

As Peggy Parish's healing of breast cancer became known more sufferers sought her husband's help. Personally and by mail the calls for healing increased. The healer went into homes and hospitals, indeed wherever there was a plea for help. His colleagues at work noticed his changed habits, which led to discovery of his healing gift. He took early retirement with a reduced income. At no time was he in need of money; always the supply met his requirements. Many volunteered to help deal with a growing correspondence. His wife Peggy was his close colleague. As late as of this writing she, in her 80's, was still healing, many years after Billy's passing.

The Parish couple lived then in a small apartment; the best room became a sanctuary in which the healer secluded himself twice daily to commune with the spirit doctors who guided his development. Billy did not ask seekers for their medical histories. He did not solicit patients. Their problems led them to his door. His knowledge of medicine and anatomy was minimal.

Gradually his psychic gifts developed. He became a trance medium, which appears to be a required stage for certain unfolding. He became almost a recluse apart from receiving patients. I recall with pleasure, after so many years, visiting his small house—and wondering why that gift had come to him and not to others. I still wonder. They must be chosen before birth.

What, you may ask, is the evidence that Parish, or others, are in contact with identified spirit entities? It is not faith that caused him to devote his life to healing but knowledge; faith followed. Parish's psychic gifts grew until clairvoyantly he saw his spirit guides. Other mediums also described them.

While working in his garden he clairvoyantly saw a man and asked his name. The spirit preferred to be called only Brother William. Parish pressed for evidence. The reply: "Go to the Royal Ophthalmic Hospital". This Parish did, finding a portrait of a former president of the hospital.

Another spirit was identified as Abdul Latif, a Persian physician whom Parish contacted through another medium for diagnostic purposes. Some 17 years earlier Abdul Latif had told an inquirer that details establishing his identity would be found in the British Museum. Search was sterile until a librarian, an eminent Orientalist, guided the inquirer to references of the noted Persian who lived some 750 years before, in the time of Richard the First of England.

Abdul Latif, the spirit, was found to have an encyclopedic knowledge of medicine, including modern dietetics, osteopathy and homeopathy. He gave Parish many proofs of his presence. As he developed the healer had less need to consult other mediums, which is a process common among those who advance as they serve.

Parish gave freely of his energy to all who sought him. He did not charge a fee. When funds were required to meet the expenses involved in the growing service by mail, they were found. His needs never became a burden, his faith in his inspirers was firm.

As in the case of Edwards, many patients saw Parish at their bedsides during absent healing, thus establishing out of the body consciousness as a highly favourable condition in healing for reasons explained in the Edwards section. In addition, Parish frequently described the rooms he visited during out of the body healings.

It should not be taken as a gospel that all healers develop as though they were of one mould, since each is different. The spirit guides take into account all the variables and work to reach conditions in which spirit energies can be transmitted to those who suffer.

In the three healers we are reviewing it is clear to me that they were chosen in advance of their birth and carefully brought forward to a condition in which their spirit mentors could not only transmit healing power through them but also make themselves and their teaching known.

I am confident that human personality is a major factor in developing a healing medium. Some of us prefer the close contact of others in all we do; a few prefer, if they can manage it, to work, as they believe, alone. It all depends upon the nature of the bond between us and our invisible guides. Much also depends upon the degree of co-operation and our responses to spirit influence.

In the three classic cases there is evidence of a relationship between the incarnate and the spirit so close that even in the "normal" state of consciousness the personality of a spirit guide emerges, sometimes in a quirk of pronunciation, sometimes in a tone of voice. That, and other evidence, tends to prove what I call the porous nature of our physical, psychic and spirit makeup. We are not secondary, nor even tertiary identities, but wonderfully complex personalities with many facets.

For Parish the later years of his life manifested these conditions and he became in a real sense a prisoner of his healing. This arose from the limits either that he imposed on himself or those established by the invisibles so that he could fulfil his mission.

I knew Billy well during his healing years. He set himself a method of serving that precluded social life. When we enjoyed an occasional day together, we were alone. He talked mainly of healing, his face radiant. We walked in lovely Richmond Park to which a private entrance had been provided by a benefactor who built him a healing sanctuary in gratitude for the healing of her husband. We did not speak of politics (I was then a political journalist) nor of the controversies that were my daily diet.

He lived by and for the spirits and his patients.

In his presence there was a peace of the kind I found later with Edwards. I suppose it is what my spirit friends call a part payment for service rendered. We each are paid as labourers worthy of our hire. Billy did not, after a while, leave his home since he had set hours for concentration on healing; between seven and eight in the morning and ten and eleven at night.

From his viewpoint Parish was following, perhaps unconsciously, the ingrained habits of western mankind which is bound to blocks in many activities and cannot readily abandon such a rhythm. For example, when he ventured from his sanctuary for a social visit, he would withdraw from conversation to concentrate on his absent patients. Even that concession to modern habits was abandoned as he withdrew from the mainstream of daily living.

So, observing out of love for a great man and healer, it has lessons now and for times to come when healing will be seen and employed in light of the gathering experience on a massive scale. As you will see in the report and study of the Edwards mission, the clock does not govern and concentration is not the means of directing the healing energies. Time is not a factor to the healing spirits.

It is almost humiliating to admit that in all my years of experience in psychical and healing activities I did not pause long enough to ask: how is the non-physical energy developed? Is it a constant, is it "produced" to meet need and demand? What agency moves the healing force or forces? We have assumed nothing in this matter since it did not occur to us that more than the immediate act of applying healing is involved.

We did not ask the appropriate questions, therefore, the enlightening answers are not given. It appears to be a spirit policy, even a rule, that unless we seek we shall not be told. In this we are not different from the scientist or any other in using the mind to increase knowledge. It is a pet theory of mine (and I like paradox) that the answer suggests the question: in short, knowledge is everywhere—if we can find it. We did not ask the questions on the mode of transfer of healing energy or of the transfer directly at the moment of a request.

So much awaits us in healing that none may fear to find a limit to it. We will not become "instant" masters of the hidden wisdom but more aware as healers and teachers.

We do know, from experience, that in some cases healing is begun before the healer receives the request, as by mail. A good question is: how is it done? We can envision an organisation so vast and efficient that it responds to requests in many nations at the same time.

Spiritualists should recall that they are not alone in the healing arts. There are others, even though they do not ascribe the source of healings to the same cause as we do. Healing is healing even if healers differ.

We know that spirit healing is not achieved by an act of the medium's will, nor by sheer power of concentration. If concentration is the answer, why does not concentration cure all? Certainly, spirit healing, or spirit healers, do not cure all. We have some way to go before we begin to understand even the mechanics of healing.

All of these thoughts were prompted by reporting Parish's method of preparing himself for healing. Not only did his concept of the need to concentrate at certain hours limit his activities but it now appears that it was necessary that his system should be tried to the limit.

How Parish came to employ absent healing I did not discover in many discussions. I have now to assume these factors contributed his awareness of distant healing in his efforts to help his wife in her being cured of cancer, his awareness of like healing as told in the Bible, and his experience in concentrating on patients at a distance while he was away from home on his duties in the railroad industry.

It soon became clear that the modern wonder of communication by mail and telephone brought more healing to more people than by any other method through all of history. How many did the Nazarene heal in his slow movement through ancient Israel? The record is not available. The effect is history. Modern spirit healers achieve more and appear to cover a wider range of cures. That may be so because we have invented more and more varied diseases by our foolish abuse of nature and ourselves.

This fact remains: Parish was the modern innovator of healing at a distance on a large scale.

I have recorded elsewhere that Parish healed me when a doctor said my survival was "between God and myself". This is written some 40 years later—a long reprieve. The distant healing process was developing then and is, I theorise, a physical replica of what occurs in the spirit realm where there is said to be no obstacle to direct, immediate verbal or non-verbal communication.

The same factors existed in the Parish healing mission as later developed in the Edwards healing: the numbers and range of diseases dealt with successfully increased. There is one exception. After some initial public healings Parish served by mail and in his sanctuary.

It was during this period I knew him best. We

exchanged many confidences and talked of our meeting to come in the spirit world. There was between us a love that sought nothing and we comforted one another that when the years of trial were over we would resume our lives together. I felt I had known him elsewhere.

Billy returned to my wife and I when we lived in the United States. He spoke in the direct voice with Frank Decker as the medium. He greeted my wife who had served him well during his closing days on earth. In two loving words Billy identified himself—and was gone.

Parish had none of the scientific curiosity of Edwards. His nature was that of the devotee. His life was service to many, so many, that at one count, he had given healing to some 500,000 whose requests came by mail.

Before giving instances of the Parish healings I must report that he idealised that beloved spirit, Silver Birch, who counselled him. Beyond that, he yearned to meet the Nazarene of whom the guide spoke to him as one deeply involved in the spread of knowledge of man's inner nature.

Frank Decker, the physical medium who invited the harsh and unfair tests of psychic researchers, visited the Parish sanctuary at East Sheen and knelt in prayer. This, he told me, was the only time he had done so. Why, I asked. He did not answer.

I am convinced that the Parish mediumship, as is the Edwards mediumship, is part of a concerted plan for human betterment in the short run and for spiritual regeneration in the long run. It is also clear to me that even their modes of healing are the expression of a progressive plan. Let us look at some evidence.

It seems self-serving to quote an article I wrote in *Psychic News* of June 13, 1942, but it follows sequentially in this narrative. This excerpt could stand for much of the Parish healing.

Harold James Blunt, of Torquay, for 50 years suffered

a contracted joint in his right foot. He sought healing from Parish. After some 10 months of absent healing, he wrote:

'It is with a very grateful heart that I write you with regard to a deformity to my right foot. I am more than pleased to say that by means of your assistance and mediumship, and the power of almighty God, the contracted joint has yielded to your wondrous gifts and has now become completely cured."

That letter was one of many selected at random, unopened, from one mail delivery. Appeals by letter for healing increased so much that the postal service made extra deliveries.

Here is another:

"It is with great joy that I write to tell you of the wonderful blessing that my brother has received. Every day he gains strength and is now able to stand upright and walk a little. He is able to take food and is gaining weight. He seems to radiate joy. After visiting him his friends say, 'It has done me good to be with him'. Doctors marvel at his progress." Other members of that family "join in thanksgiving and praise to God for this great gift".

That article remarked that as the Parish healing developed, responses from patients changed. I added ". . . as he (Parish) grows so does the quality of the response he evokes from the sufferer. It seems to me to throw light on the meaning of the statement by a spirit guide that it is impossible to heal unless you touch the souls of those who suffer".

In the course of many years of association with Parish I noticed the sincerity and emotion in letters of gratitude. Many wrote in a poor hand, the sentences were not carved in classic prose. Those who had been healed, or the relatives who wrote for them, needed no art or artifice to communicate, hence this letter:

"Words fail me, Mr. Parish, when I try to express my gratitude to you. I was in the greatest pain and agony for months, but thanks to the mercy of God, and the great power he has given you, I feel stronger now and in better health and I have done for some considerable time. The growth I had seemed to just melt away, and my pain vanished, as it were, all in such a short time."

A mother wrote:

"Now for the good news in regard to my daughter. Eight weeks ago she was advised by a specialist and doctors to enter a hospital to undergo an operation to have a polypus removed which was causing haemorrhage and obstruction. After getting in touch with you the haemorrhage ceased."

Surgery was delayed for some weeks then re-scheduled. The mother wrote:

"She (the daughter) was even placed on the operating table when the specialist decided to give her another examination and, to his amazement, found the polypus had disappeared and that there was no need for an operation to take place. The doctor said, 'This is something wonderful'."

Three days later the girl was discharged from hospital.

In capsule form, this is the core of other letters, all from the same delivery. I opened the letters:

A man fell, injuring his back so seriously he feared he would not recover. He wrote: "Now I am quite well (as a result of healing)." His wife added: "He has made a wonderful recovery. The doctors cannot understand, and say nature has been very kind to him."

Very kind indeed.

There is some evidence to show us as we truly are.

One patient developed heart trouble, his legs swelled, he became nearly blind. He wrote:

"Three doctors in succession gave me up as hopeless. I am happy to say today I can get about by myself. My only concern now is that imperfect hearing should be restored."

There is the case of the woman of 72 who had a broken wrist and arm. Her daughter wrote:

"The doctors are amazed at the way the bones have knitted together, especially at the age of 72. The doctor was commenting on this to the students (at the hospital) the last day my mother was there. She said she simply had to say she knew she had been getting spiritual healing. Naturally, the doctor had very little to say on the matter."

In each bundle of letters I handled there was at least one instance of a spirit visit by Parish to the patient and of the impressive recovery that follows, as this instance shows:

The correspondent wrote of a friend ". . . whom I put on your absent healing list . . . He informs me the first night he was on your list he was awakened by a terrible pain. He says it was like someone drawing a lump from his neck, right down his chest. The next morning the lump was gone. His doctor says there is no need for an operation. It must be a great solace to you to get such marvellous results."

Of healing there is no end in this world as it is. The letters pour in wherever a healer is raised up by the spirit. The story, in a sense, is told in one mother's letter:

"I feel I must thank you once again for your wonderful absent healing for my son. I cannot find words to express how thankful I am."

Neither can I.

It always happens when telling the healing story: you determine when enough has been told of one healer, you think a representative group of healings has been described, then, like the poet wandering in a field of wild flowers at the height of their blooming, the eye catches another, and another, until his arms are filled and he has to let go. This is the final flower of this portion of the Parish healings. I am reluctant to leave him.

A woman wrote seeking healing for a younger woman friend, crippled for many years:

"It happened quite suddenly . . . I have a glorious piece of news now. You remember about a year ago a family I am interested in named Butt got in touch with you through my persuasion? The husband was in the army and was in a dreadful state of nerves. He had terrible pain in one leg and lameness. He got quite well.

"He was so glad to be well that he and I persuaded his sister, who has been a helpless cripple for years, to communicate with you. She has had 28 operations and was in a worse condition each time.

"This poor woman couldn't walk at all, according to the hospitals, specialists and the rest. They said she would never walk again. She was a hopeless case, in fact. Well, through you she is healed. The family are overjoyed and so am I. I am, in fact, so happy that I can't even write without trembling. Our local paper is full of it because the family is well known and the case was generally regarded as hopeless.

"It happened quite suddenly, it seems. She got up without help, and for a while felt a great pain in her back, and then felt the blood in her flowing through her veins—and walked into the house. She then walked round to her sister's to prove her healing. She knows it is a 'miracle', and says so, and is grateful for having been led to you to link her up with God in this way."

Among my many convictions derived from study, experience and direct awareness of the reality of spirit existence and in the power of evolved spirits to lead and guide those who co-operate with them is this: That the years of healing covered by the three healers named here, Jones, Parish and Edwards, is the golden age of modern Spiritualism. I trust that this has been more or less clearly stated.

That does not mean that the spirit world has retired from evolution, that the spirits we know best have returned, or will soon return, to the life beyond which they enjoyed as the fruits of their service. And leave us bereft of teaching, guidance and healing?

Shall we like others who have known spirit contact fall into the gross error of contriving a testament to replace a living reality, shall we replace mediums with priests and truths with dogmas?

Not so. The emphasis on healing by one man or by one woman, with their colleagues, appears to be in a wave of change. The healing message has spread into millions of homes in Britain alone. And there is a world beyond.

The leaven of the spirit works in the bread of life to give sustenance. Our mission is not to whisper experience but to trumpet truth, not to dispute over words but to spread the great and good tidings which all mankind must in time receive as their spiritual heritage.

Those who know should not fear that the ending of one era is the tolling bell of time. An era moves to a close, a revolution in thought and action begins.

It has been and is a great privilege to live and strive in this enterprise to demonstrate how noble mankind may become. A slight increase in man's spiritual awareness would of itself constitute a revolution of such force and effect that generations hence will measure our acts and motives and declare with pride: These were our mothers and our fathers and the heritage they bequeathed us was good. Upon that we will build.

That is one man's view of a magnificent historical event, which historians may ponder far in the future.

It is said in one chronicle telling of the execution by

sword of the man who became the instrument of the Nazarene's mission that when the record of that event was inscribed it read: "A dull day; nothing happened". That nothing and what impelled it changed the world.

It cannot be said of the little band of servants of the spirit that they, too, achieved nothing; they changed thought and religion which together contribute most of mankind's motivations.

Is that nothing?

And so I say of myself and of this work: it is a privilege to have been a scribe of so much and an honour to have served with those who defamed none, who shed no blood, waged no war, gathered little of the world's goods but brought the spirit again before mankind so that a choice might be made: to seek spirit truth and, finding it, to live in its benign and creative light or to persist in ignorance of a divine heritage which is theirs.

Edwards—A Signpost
In Development of
Spirit Healing

Healer/Medium
Who Carried New
View of Man to
The Public

Absent Healing—Out
of the Body Healing

Discarnate Minds Source
Of Healing—Not the
Subconscious Mind

Doctors Healed

## HARRY EDWARDS

All movements are but the lengthened reflections of one man, or woman, or of a small band of pioneers. The Spiritualist-based healing movement of the last 130 years is such; it has no head or chief in the world, its inspiration is of the spirit; hence no man or group of men and women control or direct either the selection of its demonstrations or advocates.

With each phase of development a band of enthusiasts soon gathers about a sensitive person showing some aspect of the psychic and spiritual gifts. So unstructured and disestablished is this movement that it has, as yet, no satisfactory historical records. Historians have neglected it although the subject is recorded throughout history. There is no evidence of any mysterious restriction on the writing of such a history; the effort was made once by Sir Arthur Conan Doyle. He was more successful with Sherlock Holmes. That sole effort at a history of Spiritualism is unsatisfactory. There is no single comprehensive library, no single collection of physical documents available as research material for a history; and no museum of artifacts, nor of spirit-inspired art. Fortunately, there is an array of newspapers, books, pamphlets which may one day be assembled for the use of historians. Then it will be seen how rich and informative is the record.

And since all histories are but the records of men and women, in short, the story of mankind, we now are at the place where we review the histories, or stories, of the pioneers in the Spiritual movement. A few pioneers are selected, not at random, but of deliberate choice since they, on the evidence available, are outstanding as signposts on the soul's adventure into physical existence and, following its disciplines, its heartbreaks and joys, its failures and achievements, and its return, greater, wiser and prepared for a fuller life.

The pioneer in spirit healing, in any period, does not appear to be self-chosen. He or she, without exception, experiences great difficulty in reaching a point of decision to serve. Not all who begin complete the course; many fall away for a variety of reasons. Their decisions are easy to understand for the pressure on a potential medium is severe. Indeed, the measure of achievement is the measure of endurance. This, in part, explains how healer/mediums become aware of their gifts, how they are developed, how they begin to serve and what they again endure at that stage of development as at all others. The process does not end until we are free of the obligation undertaken before coming to earth.

As the pioneer sets the signposts as he moves forward the role is more difficult since it involves, generally, the public life, controversy, frequently abuse and, on occasion, persecution. Surely no one would knowingly set out on such a course if fully aware of the consequences—unless there were prior knowledge somewhere in the consciousness. Predestination? Not as the philosophers have it but as a matter of choice before birth when the decision is made knowingly.

Without specifying any one healer/medium as belonging to such a band of volunteer missionaries, we can for the purpose of the healing story select Harry Edwards as the third of the band responsible for a clearly defined period of development in spiritual healing which now gives way to what I claim is a Democracy of Spirit Healing. The others are, Fred Jones and Billy Parish.

Like the other two, Edwards served in the area centred on London. Unlike the others he is a public figure. Jones was hedged about by the sheer numbers he treated daily under the influence of his healing guide, Medicine Man.

Edwards was the beneficiary of the efforts of his two predecessors. Jones and Parish, in the sense that in his person he took to the public forum the art of spirit healing in a manner that had not before been achieved. Of course, there were others. They, too, contributed to the growing areas of interest. Every public meeting, each so-called exposure, all clerical warnings as to the alleged but never proved dangers, and all misreporting by the popular press did not stay the interest. By the time the Church of England, for example, had reluctantly agreed to an inquiry into Spiritualism, it was much too late for any opposition to succeed. That the Church of England's Commission of Inquiry into Spiritualism reported favourably is an historic fact; that it saw in Spiritualism a hope of reviving interest in Christianity is a fact—which it also ignored, to its loss.

The next church commission of inquiry—into what it called Divine Healing—did not lead to so fundamental an admission. The clerical priests had found an ally in the medical priests. But in both the church and in medicine were, and are, men and women who will not be told what to believe. The yeast was at work. Opinion in medicine and in the church in favour of personal involvement in spiritual healing is a fact, and neither the Church of England nor the British Medical Association can prevent the invisible spirit from finding its way into the minds and hearts of those who are moved towards spiritual things.

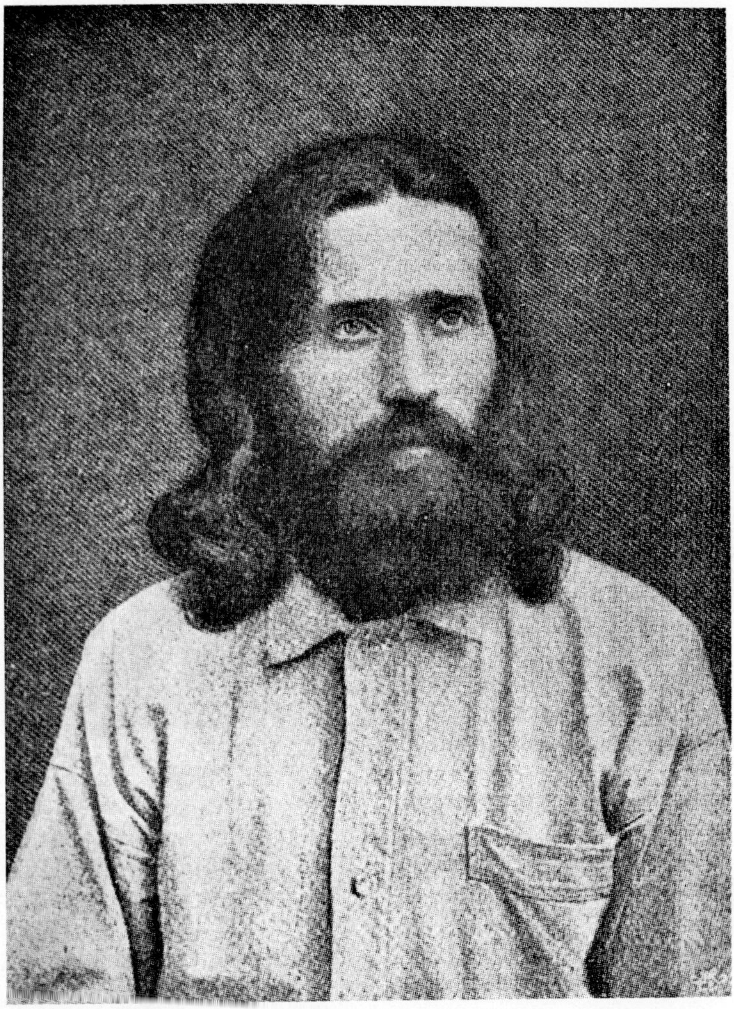

FRANCIS SCHLATTER

Mystery Man Schlatter appeared in a Colorado U.S. city without contacts, healed hundreds daily by laying on hands, did not take fees, lived an ascetic life, became the focus for thousands of the sick – and the dishonest. His departure was as mysterious as his arrival. He left his hosts a simple note: his Father, he stated, had called him away.

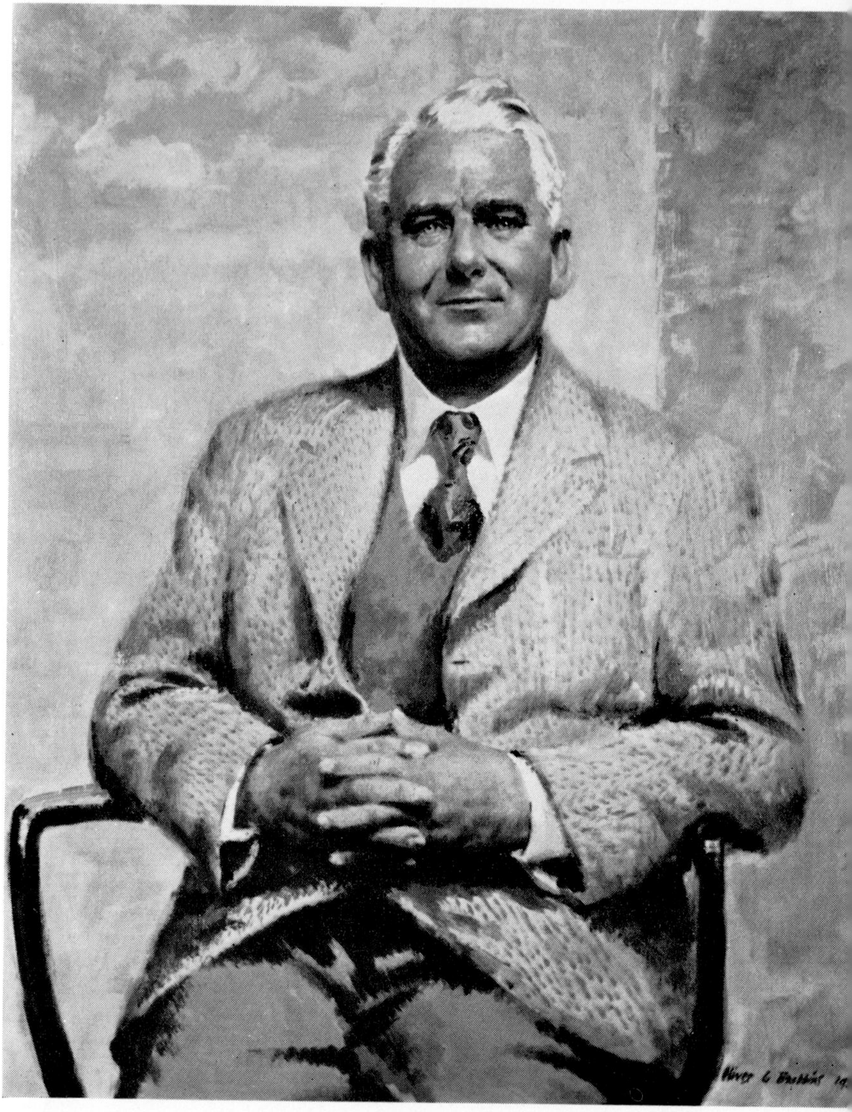

HARRY EDWARDS, A PORTRAIT

He advanced spirit healing to heights never before achieved and is today the outstanding healer in the world. He simplified concepts of healing. His fearless defence of the healing mission encouraged thousands to try to follow where he led. One of his goals is to advance healing as a natural activity expressing a spiritual force with least human-imposed limitations.

I have before me a personal letter from the Rev. Maurice Elliott, a veritable Daniel in this matter, opening his heart on the difficulties he faced in persuading the Church of England leaders even to inquire into the question of Survival. Is it not strange that a church founded upon Survival should be urged to prove for itself what it professes to believe? Elliott lost much in preferment by his courageous advocacy; he also helped many in and out of the church to gain new hope based on fact.

These instances of widespread efforts to influence public opinion at all levels: the personal, the scientific, the literary, the hearing of massive proof of Survival at large public meetings—all culminated, as I said elsewhere, in the death of Helen Duncan, the remarkable materialisation medium, and in the triumph of the Edwards mission. That says nothing yet of the role of a tiny group of journalists and authors who filled the historic role of scribes, for as a Chinese sage has said: Palest ink is stronger than strongest memory.

Edwards, who has reached the peak of his mission and now in patient dignity serves as always had, like the others, a humble beginning. He was born in London in 1893, one of a family of nine. His father was a typesetter. Harry was apprenticed to his father's trade. His first duty, in the caste system of those days, was as floor sweeper. His own account, given me in preparing his early biography, was of a positive character: from printing, which he disliked, to a passion for politics as a remedy for what ailed Britain in those days. The basic needs remain, only the pattern and the antagonists change, in name only. The healer/medium, although he may not always be aware of it, is a true reformer in that he provides a substantial reason for healing, personal and social, as an essential to the fuller life of spirits in the flesh.

Our future healer found his voice as protestant against the obvious wrongs in society—and in those areas of London that so shocked the famous, but now almost forgotten American novelist-reformer, Jack London. Jack London also had his psychic baptism; his mother was a medium. The literary critics do not like that fact and show it.

Edwards had a good education at the University of Adversity which was widely attended by millions of British citizens of that day. The university is still in business. It is one of the aims of spirit teaching that that awful monument to man's inhumanity to man be closed permanently for lack of students. He served in World War I, in the Middle East and in India, where his dislike of printing as a career had its wry side: he became editor of a battalion magazine waging there the same kind of campaign he had been developing in helping to right social wrongs in the London area.

He saw colonialism at work, he saw the awful sores of Middle East poverty; the degradation of women who were the victims of the degradation of their men. And he observed the greater dignity and humanity of the women. Our future healer did as much as he could to ameliorate the woes of oppressed peoples. Bangalore, India, or a lonely post on the Indian North-West frontier were different only in degree from the East End of London. He saw the fire worshippers and the devil dancers, the greedy public officials and the general decay which is always produced by corruption and lack of respect of men for one another. He was friend to the oppressed and occasionally the healer of the sick. At his departing from his post as British Army Director of Labour, with 250,000 men, women and children under his control, "the road he knew so well was lines of weeping people crying, 'You are our father and our mother, do not leave us' ".

Edwards' life for the following 20 years was an unremitting struggle against debt. At one point he set a record of 18 court warrants for debt. Even the court marshals became his friends. The printer who hated printing had not lost his political reforming zeal; a therapy against business woes. The world, he was sure, could be helped by the new League of Nations. His community could be helped by his presence in Parliament. He graduated from direct participation in politics as a result of the 1935 general election. By his destiny he attracted tests. He was an anti-printing printer; he was not a successful businessman; his final effort as a politican was made in a London constituency, North-West Camberwell Green.

He lost the election and his deposit; he had trouble getting transportation home where he and his wife (she with a blistered foot) found that some laundry left drying had been singed. The Edwards' sought to console themselves with hot cocoa. He lifted his cup. The bottom fell out. His political career was ending. Some time later he learned to read such clear, powerful messages not as proof of defeat but as earnest of a change in direction.

How does a medium or a healer/medium become aware of potential? The paths followed by so many of them are so similar that it appears there is almost a standard practice manual in the spirit world. At Ilford in Essex as an amateur conjurer and member of a group of magicians, he decided to visit a Spiritualist church to detect what he thought was trickery. He was not clear about the clairvoyant message given by a medium but he was impressed. In 1934, he joined a development circle at a Spiritualist church in his neighbourhood. In time, he said, he "felt the rhythm of his body quickening, breathing became faster, his mind was dominated by a single thought he desired to express, but he could not speak because his throat would not respond to his will".

He was forced to stand up. The desire to speak was so strong that he cried out in a loud voice, "Let peace come to all people". His explanation then was that his mind was filled with thoughts of peace movements and anti-war speeches.

His explanation is that "it may well have been that his subconscious reactions were used by the spirit people to promote mediumship under some form of spirit possession through some domination of his subconscious mind".

This aspect of Edwards' development shows that already he had touched on the explanation of the process of spirit control, or influence, by the subconscious mind.

In a following experience through his lips came speech in another voice not his own while in a trance state, and expressing ideas he had not thought out, and in phrasing different from his own. He later had visions; in a supernormal state he saw the unregenerate in their struggles contrasted with liberated, happy people. Edwards' views of these experiences shook his rationalist outlook and moved his basic concept from the national to the universal. His public speaking improved as spirit control became closer. He had not been a praying man but under spirit influence he referred to biblical passages he had not read. Prayer-like utterances became easier. He was always aware of what was being said, which is not uncommon. He was persuaded another intelligence was using his faculties, an entity, an American Indian whose name, White Feather, was given by another medium.

He had other mediumistic experiences which persuaded him of the reality of spirit control. As a test of that reality he decided to inject one of his own thoughts into an address to be given through him. He planned to be sure that if the guide failed he, Edwards, could speak. From my book, *Born to Heal*, this is quoted: "He allowed his mind to be controlled, he heard his phrases being uttered. Then everything stopped. He could not even utter the platitudes used on all platforms to fill gaps made by lapses of memory." The orator sat down, the meeting was spoiled—but his experiment proved to him that he was controlled for the addresses.

All of that is a lesson in spirit control and in co-operation by the medium: it was also a preparation for the healing mission, intimations of which now suffused his mind. It also teaches of the processes of gradual development of co-operation to reach a point at which the long-range project of healing could begin. That example alone should teach aspirants that the way to initiation into service is long and difficult; that endurance is the essential quality for without it none of the rest will emerge. It also shows the patience and skill of the entities who must gain some measure of control of the medium before he reaches the level of inspiration.

Again, the future healer's psychic nature which includes his nervous system has to be attuned, or become capable of attunement, to the subtle and intricate spirit direction of healing forces. This shows intelligence of the highest order, planning and foresight—all in a philanthropic venture of co-operation. How else could Edwards—and the others—become so sensitive to spirit influence unless they had undergone the long training and attunement required? He had learned how to relax and become controlled; he had learned also to control the controlling phase. This also is a requisite to the disciplined psychic life; not to permit what is not desired. It also shows that this power to decline is equal to the power to assent and draws attention to other aspects of co-operative healing, such as absent treatment; I mean by that a flexibility and response to spirit influence of the kind operating through the healer's subconsciousness when he is in the waking state and when he is asleep—a revelation for any psychologists and psychiatrists who care to study that phenomenon.

The views of those who have not experienced the phases of mediumistic development are bizarre when they theorise, without basis in fact, about split personalities, extensions, hallucinations and the like. If results in healing are a criterion, then the healer/mediums have outstanding success while the ratio of success to treatment in the psychological and psychiactric field is minor by comparison. Not only are such successes minor by comparison but they are achieved more slowly and are minimal by comparison. When we move the analysis from the complex, non-physical treatment of psychology and psychiatry to the spirit healing, it has to be said that the difficulties are much greater for the orthodox practitioners who do not have the spirit co-operation which could transform their capability to heal. That day will come, but not until there has been a clearer understanding by psychologists and psychiatrists of the reality, nature and power of spirit healing and of the necessity of following the same development as is required to bring out the latent capabilities in a healer/medium of, say, the Edwards level.

It is unlikely that we are on what is called a straight line path of development; that is to say that from the Edwards achievement all who come after will be of like nature and readiness to co-operate and more successful. I do not think that the next stage will be but a continuation of the one now at its peak. For example, we in the flesh do not understand how to recognise which person will become a healer and which one will not. We do not yet know how to evaluate the potential of any psychic instrument. Even where that is known by the directing spirits, we as yet have not developed the insight required to show whether the potential healer will persist—the hardest part.

We have already followed Edwards' tracks along the psychic way; we know the physical facts; we do not know of the inner development. There is a project worthy of philanthropic support.

At some point this phase of the work has to be begun because the total of healers is rising. In such a situation there must be standards of achievement, a code of ethics, some reliable means of evaluation and a counselling service to advise healers who are aware of a need.

There is no call for rigid controls of the kind found in the orthodox healing arts. These have controls that maintain power, a legal sanction over training, conduct and discipline, the closed circles of a privileged few. We have to look to a Democracy of Healing knowing well that where power is diffused it may also be diluted. This is not to assert there is an automatic danger of abuse of power; the reverse is true, for the power to heal does not rest with or reside in us: it emanates from the spirit and may and would be withdrawn where the conduct of the instrument fell below the requirements for spirit co-operation. It is as simple as that. The power to license, say, a physician, is held by his peers who are reluctant to condemn. Where a medium falls below the spirit standard, the power is withdrawn, the inspiration fails and woefully at times, artifice supplies what discipline and inspiration alone can perform. When the medium fails to deliver, the earnest seeker withdraws. It is, in a sense, analogous to the law of the market place, with control in the hands of the spirit.

All of these are considerations in retelling part of the Edwards saga for a new generation is here. Such considerations must arise because of the importance of the subject. We again take Edwards' development as an example because of his long experience and skill in analysing not only his own situation but in teaching that where he has been others may follow and excel.

Our healer/medium has been through the phases of influence, control, trance speaking, visions and now is at the point of launching on the mission for which he was prepared by a life of hardship, frustration and failure that did not in any way deteriorate his cheerful, buoyant nature—all required for healing since we all influence the power that flows through us to others.

Edwards' initial desire to heal was curbed by his self-consciousness, a psychological state well marked in emerging mediums; also, it is a sign of humility. In addition he was aware of other invisible personalities about him.

Among his direct personal experiences was one in which he was hurled bodily across the gap between himself and an oncoming vehicle—"lifted up and hurled across the gap", is his expression. People who saw the incident were astonished. They said so. On another occasion when he and a friend were in a car on a quiet suburban street, the friend braked abruptly and switched off the engine. As he did so a heavy horse-drawn vehicle sped in front of the stopped car and came to rest in a garden. Edwards and his friend wondered how the incident happened, especially about the motor being stopped. Their conclusion: spirit intervention.

His first experience of absent healing developed when he tried absent healing, then becoming widely known through the successes of Billy Parish. Edwards was told of someone suffering from tuberculosis, pleurisy and haemorrhage. As he began silent treatment he visualised a hospital ward and focused on one bed, "saw" the patient clearly and said so to the woman who had asked for healing on behalf of the sick person. She confirmed the details. When Edwards told me of that incident many years ago he said that he could clearly recall the incident. He knew then that intense efforts were being made to arouse awareness of the healing power. He was informed that the sick man's recovery began the night Edwards began treatment, remember at a distance. Fever lessened, bleeding stopped, pleurisy ceased. In one week the recovering man was out of danger and was sent to a sanatorium. He recovered fully and returned to work.

I like to think that Edwards, for his initial effort, was shown a vision of the hospital ward in which lay the first person to be healed as an evidence of spirit knowledge of what occurs when absent healing is given. Edwards has had many out of the body experiences in which he has been seen by some who had either sought healing or for whom healing had been sought by others. It is an example also of how spirit healers work. They know from the appeal for the healer's service who is in need, where located, condition, and upon spirit examination, the remedy to be applied. Having once seen one segment of the process so early in his career, his later experiences filled in the rest of the picture. Because of his service, Edwards was shown the process, a procedure that would not necessarily be repeated. That one experience was for instruction and assurance. Just as he had, for a time, given trance addresses which convinced him of the existence of spirit guides and of their ability to influence his mind in order to help others, it was not required to do so every time he gave healing. The lesson learned, the faculty to heal was increased and improved. Visions were no longer required.

The Edwards records are so filled with cures of every kind of disease that to select one or some, or few or many, becomes difficult for repetitions become repetitious until only a statistical abstract will tell the healing story. From one cure at a distance to some 15,000,000 requests for healing in 45 years is a modern wonder. It is satisfying for me, at least, to know that so much blessed relief has come to this world through the pioneering efforts of one man.

I am aware that he has loyal colleagues and supporters. But he had to begin somewhere after a long and arduous apprenticeship. The beginning must have been planned.

The first healing was a test of both healer and his spirit collaborators; tuberculosis, pleurisy, haemorrhage. The next of a man with lung cancer. The wife wrote Edwards a long, detailed letter, the substance being that the husband resumed work prematurely following influenza. Family problems induced shock and weight loss and finally cancer—a model case for the healer's later view that cancer can be caused by emotional and mental stress. A specialist's report advised that the patient be made "comfortable", the usual roundabout method of predicting death. The wife, despondent, on a Sunday evening walk felt a strong urge to enter a Spiritualist church. She was surprised to find Edwards was the speaker whom she had known but had not seen for some years. A few days later the wife, Mrs. N., was surprised to find Edwards in a store while shopping in the ordinary way. She told him of her anxiety over her husband's illness. The husband's name was added to the list for a following meeting at the Spiritualist church. Mrs. N. wrote: "My husband naturally knew nothing of this because it was not intended he should. In his bad nervous condition this was not to be thought of, and as he was an agnostic he would have laughed at the whole affair. However, during the night he became so much better that he got up quite early in the morning, announcing he felt remarkably well, and made an early cup of tea . . . He looked a new man. The most surprising thing was his altered complexion, and the tired look had vanished from his eyes . . . The healing had taken place on the previous day."

Mrs. N.'s letter ends: "I am convinced that the sudden, wonderful change in my husband's condition was due to the help given to him through the prayers of my Spiritualist friends."

As Edwards comments—Mr. N. did not know of his existence prior to the healing. They did not meet at any time.

That, and other early healings, are chosen because they are early, following a period of intense development and as showing that the healer was indeed launched on his career. Also, the varied nature of the ills cured show that spirit healing is an all-embracing service, that the healing follows requests, that the maladies treated are all different and serious, that it made little difference, then, whether the healing was by the distant or absent method or by contact. The superior results of absent unscheduled healing had yet to be established.

In the short sequence of events leading to Edwards' emergence as a public figure these healings occurred:

A young woman was told by a medium at a Spiritualist meeting that her sister was seriously ill and she should seek out a man named Edwards, with a directive on how to find him. The address given was inaccurate but was located through inquiries at a Spiritualist church. Late that night Edwards saw the young woman who was seeking help for her sister. He said he would call on her the following morning and would ask that night for healing. The following morning he found the sick woman's temperature near normal from 103 degrees and gave more healing. From the book, *Born to Heal*: "That afternoon the patient brought up a large mass of black matter, which so alarmed her mother that she immediately sent for a doctor, who said the patient was in a dangerous condition, too dangerous to be moved to a hospital. He ordered quiet. Blinds were drawn to ensure that not even light would disturb her."

The patient's sister told Edwards what had happened. He saw the sick woman, became aware of a feeling of calmness and happiness, comforted the mother and sister. He saw that the sick woman would be convalescent by the Sunday following. The mother was sceptical. As foretold, on the following Sunday the young woman was well enough to rise and take tea. Sometime later, the healer said, she dressed normally and walked about.

It was only after the young woman had been healed that Edwards learned she had been in a sanatorium as a result of tuberculosis, that one lung was collapsed and that she expected to have air refills for at least three years. She asked for spirit healing so that she could marry. She did not have more air refills. Her doctors, puzzled, sent her back to the sanatorium for observation. The following spring the medical superintendent of the hospital wrote to the young woman, Gladys C.: "You will be glad to know that I was entirely satisfied with your film. There is no sign whatever of the cavity now, and I think you have done remarkably well. I hope you will keep well".

Gladys C. married, had children, the tuberculosis did not recur. Nine years later she did fairly heavy work in a furniture store.

The second healing in the family was given to the younger sister who had sought out Edwards as a result of the message from a medium at a Spiritualist church. This second young woman had a foot deformed from birth and had surgery twice. It was said some small bones had been removed. Additionally a bony growth was developing between the toes. Three days after Edwards had given healing the bony growth disappeared, leaving only loose skin where the growth had been. For months healing was given; the foot strengthened, flesh formed over the skeleton-like limb until the support worn was discarded. This young woman then walked normally. During World War II she drove an ambulance, using her right foot which prior to healing was so deformed as to require the support. Among other members of the family successfully treated was the father who was cured of a cataract.

It now became clearer to the healer that the cures were not coincidental or what are called remissions; not even spontaneous, because his healing was sought by this one family and all the cures were striking. It is a fair conclusion that healers in the spirit directed the family to seek healing, since they formed a test group that would produce such results as would encourage Edwards. He concentrated on healing, his successes became known in his neighbourhood, requests for healing flowed in week by week until newspapers found he was news. One area newspaper featured his healing for three successive weeks.

The reluctant printer's life was filled with healing. He set aside one day each week for healing on his return, tired from his work in his print shop. Two rooms of his small home became what in other places—and countries, is called a temple. It was certainly a temple of healing. Edwards, with an associate, gave healing to all in the filled rooms from 10.00 to 10.30 p.m. Records of each healing were kept then, together with medical and psychic diagnoses, rate of progress, or lack of it.

As the demand for healing grew another night each week was set aside for absent healing. I believe that my friend, Billy Parish, was at least in part responsible for the word "intercession" used by him and other healers to describe the healer's action in seeking healing. In my book, *Born to Heal*, I tried to deal with that view and find no reason now, after 30 years, to change it—that we do not intercede as though pleading for something not available by request; a kind of obeisance before some lesser deity. Surely a sincere request for healing addressed in silence or spoken, or written, should be sufficient to make the contact from healer/medium to the healer in the spirit. Be that as it may, Edwards and his colleague made their requests by whatever name called—and there were responses resulting in healing at a distance, in increasing numbers.

The elements of increasing cures occurring among increasing cases was encouragement—but like factors with absent healing cures added makes a striking development. I will try to show elsewhere, in my adopted country, America, there were spirit healings just as remarkable as those of their British successors with some differences and development which will be set out. This is done, not to make the report a contest but as showing there is, as already repeatedly stated here, a long range plan directed from the spirit world for the relief and spiritual regeneration of man. The relief is in the healing; regeneration takes much longer.

Another development in the Edwards healing is that he brought the question of faith out of the mysterious place where it had been kept by theologians for many centuries. The question was—and still is—if we have faith enough it will heal the sick and, if we accept certain biblical statements it will, perhaps, remove mountains. It is not a facile reply to point out that removing a mountain is a substantial problem. I live in an area of Southern California which is in a continuous state of earthly trembling because of geological faults. One fault movement raised a portion of a mountain range some five feet in the air. No doubt an engineer could calculate the energy required to raise that mass, say, five feet. Nature has the energy. The question now is: do we humans have somewhere, concealed in our bodies or minds a secret force which when actuated by an attitude of mind called faith, however defined, will remove mountains? I doubt that but add: the position is taken here that a request for healing is a movement of thought which is conveyed through the healer/medium to the healer in spirit by whom action will be taken to respond. If the conditions warrant, the healing force exerted or applied will result in a cure, an improvement, or neither. Where does faith enter? If faith is merely acceptance of a point of view lacking knowledge of the forces or natural laws involved, then we have no need of healers; a simple request, even an intercession will do, if you have the correct attitude.

It was Edwards who first drew my attention to the faith problem, which emerged in an exchange of views on absent healing. In this section of this work, you have the first case reported of Edwards' healing in which the wife of the very sick man stated she would not tell her husband; he was an agnostic and would laugh at the idea. I doubt a man so sick would laugh at anything. The point is: he could not have faith, agnostic or firm believer, because he did not know of the healing effort on his behalf. Therefore, whose was the faith? That faith is a constituent in thought, emotion and action is obvious, else we could not take one step after another. But such faith is a path followed as a result of a prior thought expressed and finding such response that it means what St. Paul said: To your faith add knowledge, because faith is the substance of what we hope will come to pass: every thought as action will achieve it.

Leaving questions of faith, intercession and others aside, there is a further consideration: concentration. This is raised now since the concept of a thought focused on a subject bringing about a desired result is not new; indeed it is as natural as daylight. When Edwards in his early period as healer met with a group to give absent treatment, the names of patients, their locations and diagnoses were read out. There is a refreshing air of naïveté in this, as seen following many years of service. I mean that these most earnest seekers acted as though the spirit healers had to be informed vocally of sick people's names, locations and diseases. Concentration would begin and any observations made during the effort noted. Letters following such efforts would be scrutinised for clues as to the efficacy of the concentration; it seemed to be the aim of the healing group to speed the healing force on its way to the suffering applicants for healing. It is easy to see that such a method long continued would be self-defeating because of its time-consuming demands.

Edwards now holds, with many experiences and successes to support his belief, that concentration inhibits healing, since concentrating produces tension. It is easy to demonstrate his claim—and my belief, since in the absence of concentration, as in the patient's sleep, cures are achieved more rapidly and more frequently. So, we acquire another concept while we are building a rationale not only to explain, and hopefully teach, part of the art of becoming a healer, but to explain how the teaching developed—by direct personal experience, the best and lasting method.

In time the detailed record-keeping was dropped because it had served its purpose. Other factors emerged in the course of experience. Those readers with much experience in this field will, of course, recognise that this section is, as it is intended to be, a restatement, with additional matter, of much that appeared in *Born to Heal* and in some of Edwards' own writings. This is done because a whole new generation has grown up since the original books were published. While the continuous publication of cases and cures has had its own value, the point of interest is blunted by continuous repetition of the same kind of material. The purpose of this work is, as said, to demonstrate intelligence, planning and progressive direction. By capsulating the early and later developments of outstanding healers there should be an increased interest in the healing story. When you have absorbed the brief histories of pioneers preceding Edwards you will, I hope, see the case is made, completely in support of the threefold claim above. There is more than the British experience to be covered. Unfortunately there are few records of healing as we know it outside the English-speaking community. Therefore, we have to deal with the American experience which was earlier known and much recorded. There always has been some reciprocity in spiritual matters between the two nations; not as much as it should—and could have been, but still reciprocal.

Thus, when the contemporary and the historic record is read we should know why this statement developed as it did; it is intentional.

Having, for a while, left Edwards' gathering experience and skill in the art of co-operation, we find on returning to him that during the concentration periods instead of remaining concentrated he found he could travel beyond the body. His first experiences were momentary. He found himself in a patient's room. Upon realising what was happening he learned to maintain control since he had conscious awareness of being elsewhere other than in his bed for some seconds. Letters, unsought, from patients confirmed his out of the body travel. He saw patients and their visitors. In time he stopped looking for confirmation. Those who claim to have experience out of the body consciousness tell of their feelings as they travel. Edwards had no such experience.

Remarkable as is that phase of development, its purpose was limited. The gift of consciousness at a distance manifested itself when he made his mind blank and his spirit assumed control as he "photographed" an image or motion picture of the patient, the room and the health condition. As the years of development passed the healer learned he no longer sought assurance of spirit control.

The gift, so much talked and written about, was laid aside; its purpose had been served.

Of the hundreds of out of the body experiences Edwards does not recall once having taken part in a healing. Unless we can see all that occurs in a healing we cannot know the whole story. In essence it appears that the healer's role is passive. This gets rid of the magnetic passes, the "throwing away" of presumed diseased "whatever", the strokings, the heavy breathing and so on. Glamour of possession of a secret power to heal fades in the daylight of knowledge. If, as we see, Edwards did not take part directly and consciously in his beyond the body experiences, how was and how is the healing done?

Let us examine the situation: the diseased person calls for healing, or someone requests it on his behalf, with or without his knowledge. The spirit healers make the psychic, invisible contact. How? Do we, in our advanced technology of scanning and communication, have superiors in the spirit world who have known for centuries what are to us recent discoveries? How do the spirits locate the patient? I don't know unless our thought picture of the one seeking healing is a contact and that the name is a contact. But, what of the geography? Before leaving this earth, I would like to find out because the situations developed from what is usually miscalled the mystery of healing are intriguing. I surmise there are excellent reasons for Edwards not seeing nor being allowed to see the entire act of healing.

The foregoing does not even touch the question of diagnosis, nor does it approach the question of the energies involved. Then we have the question: what kind of energies are they that are directed by the will of invisible healers? Are the energies of such character that they require modification before or during application so that only the diseased cells are healed, or eliminated?

That aspect has already been treated. Is there a catalyst in the nature of the medium?

There is no report of any recipient of spirit healing having been injured in any way. The only side effects are towards improvement which continues after the initial relief.

But it is observed that as each stage of development is established, it is no longer required that the healer follow it; in a sense it would appear that the experience gathered then finds its level in the vast storehouse of the subconscious, retrievable when the need for it arises.

It is interesting to me that it was correctly forecast in 1942 that spirit healing would be developed to the point it reached some time ago—with minimal physical contact. This is the basis of the overwhelming majority of Edwards' 15,000,000 healing efforts so far. Simple arithmetic shows he could not have physically touched 15,000,000 persons in many countries, nor could he have "concentrated" on that number. There is nothing to be gained by exaggerating the numbers healed, since that would not heal anyone. There must be a vast spirit organisation at work.

It is now clear, I hope, that Edwards thought through all that he experienced, laying aside the practices followed by those who hold to ways that do not always bear rational examination. He found that by shaping his own course he was following where the increasing cures led. Each new step marked a stage of growth until today he has shed all extraneous practices and gives of himself for healing. The old concepts of hand-washing, making passes, throwing "bad vibrations" and disease aside; all these have gone since they did not, for him, withstand analysis as having any direct link with spirit healing. He had tried most of the old ways.

Even the view cherished by some that this or that colour of itself is a healing agent had to go. Healing is not achieved by colour, though psychic energies are shown by their colours. There is no question that colour is an influence on our moods and that we even choose colours subconsciously either to reflect a mood or convey an attitude. The same may be said of incense, perfume, sitting in certain positions with palms upward as though psychic energy could not just as easily flow from the back of the hand as from the palm.

These are not major matters but mention of them clears the air of misconceptions as to value of the outward signs when the truth of healing is inward and declares itself to us in slow degrees—as we approach those stages of development at which we lay aside concepts outworn for us because we must not seek refuge in bypaths.

It seems clear, to me at least, that we have gone a long way in studying healing since this story began to unfold. As Edwards' experience grew by dealing with an increasing number of patients so did his ability to describe in precise terms his convictions as to the basic facts of healing. Here is a characteristic statement on the spirit guides' ability to select which force and which degree of force to be used in a specific case:

"To achieve this there must be a directing, discarnate intelligence capable of directing and differentiating".

On the question of the role of the subconscious mind, he says:

"But whether it be healing, clairvoyance or physical activity the same answer applies: there is not any evidence that mankind possesses today, or has ever possessed, the detailed knowledge for its accomplishment and, therefore, it cannot be existent in the subconscious mind; there has been no human experience upon which this subconscious mind can draw such precise and profound wisdom. The implication follows that the directing, discarnate intelligence has been able to acquire wider knowledge than man possesses. To carry out such healings of the physical body this wisdom must not only include the employment of metaphysical forces, but the intelligence must know how to combine them with the physical forces that govern the human anatomy far in advance of our own."

Edwards adds this explanation of the mode of healing:

"Consequent of a thought appeal by a human instrument, a discarnate mind is able to receive the request and is then able to apply the correct quality of force to the particular disharmony in the body of the patient."

I add my own comment. Either the healings are achieved as Edwards says, or God has favourites.

It is fortunate that Edwards, the former printer who disliked printing, developed, along with his healing and growing awareness in other directions, a skill in writing. His output is large and his style clear. To maintain the momentum gained I attempt a condensation of his thoughts:

The healer drops all thought of mundane things. His spiritual mind takes over. Surrender is the goal, an achievement requiring much sustained discipline. Almost a paradox: surrender is the hardest psychic art by which we achieve most by doing least. Persistence brings success. Surrender becomes second nature. Another personality merges with the seeker's. Confidence and power fill his being. One thought dominates: the patient's condition.

Intrusion of other thoughts are keenly felt. The healer becomes aware of intelligence and directed movement. The mind seems to act through the fingertips—possibly the origin of the laying on of hands. This view is strengthened by the feeling of consciousness in the hands, as though the mind were at the fingertips as the healer is directed to the areas and organs in need of healing.

Intelligence rules all. Speech and movement around him seem remote; questions on the patient's condition are answered easily, by the spirit guide's greater knowledge. This is the art of becoming attuned to the spirit by yielding the body's influence. And, in his own words, the climax:

"The great joy of healing in this way is experienced when the treatment is nearing completion. The healer becomes aware of a feeling of intense pleasure, as he knows inwardly that the healing has been successful, a feeling of ecstasy that pervades his whole being."

What is summarised is the mystical experience of communion, now stated in terms most can appreciate. What for many centuries has been stated as most mysterious because cloaked in language remote and said to be religious is now told for what it is: a willing, yielding, blending of consciousness; the healer/medium by surrender raises his awareness and the guide lowers his. In such condition the healing is done.

That description by Edwards sets out the experiences in contact healing. Incidents in the patient's history are disclosed to the healer's consciousness. Incidents explaining cause of disease are traced in sufficient form to help direct the healing force. Patients forget; the subconcious remembers and reports through the healer's heightened sensitivity. The information flows, as needed, "from spirit mind to spirit mind".

Spirit healing is not an automatic service. The one desiring help, or someone desiring help for him, must initiate the healing.

In a simple anecdote Edwards tells of the illness of the wife of a friend, the medium Arnold Clare. Clare's guide was asked why she had not been helped. He replied, "We have not been asked". That night healing was requested while Clare was in trance; the cure was swift. Mrs. Clare rose next morning to meet a medical specialist who had come from London to a country hospital to encase her in plaster. The importance is stressed by Edwards and his colleague, Parish, of the patient-to-be making the first request for healing since that is proof of need and evidence of readiness to co-operate.

Another point made is that there may be many healings not recognised as being of spirit origin as a result of calls for help made by relatives, friends, doctors, clergymen and others whose silent pleas evoke spirit responses. This also depends upon the availability of others to act as catalytic agents.

This is the point at which we may summarise: Edwards' experience is given because, in my view, he is the most effective in extent, depth and numbers of healings. Experience taught him to break new ground—in this age—because the inevitable state of hardening had reached a point close to an orthodoxy, a rigidity of thought and practice. The experiences in attunement alone are beyond any stated by mystics and those who write about the subject. Mostly the writings are remote from experience.

In the case of healing of the kind done through Parish and Edwards it was achieved in conscious co-operation with spirit beings. Such an awareness is not stated by what I call the intellectual mystics who write much and do little to employ their gifts in helping humankind. They become, by choice, remote; not for them publicly-known association with spirit beings. Presumably they go directly to the Deity, or to their own unsupported notions.

Be that as it may, the fact remains that only in Spiritualism with its open avowal of the existence and direction of spirit guides are the claims of and for remotely-dwelling mystics and occultists brought into the light of public opinion. Because men of the stature of

Parish and Edwards became public figures the greater power flowed through them. What is written in many ancient and obscure scrolls, parchments and books filled with clues and metaphors, is openly taught today because the healers and all other categories of mediums are loyal to the missions they undertake.

There is not anywhere in the world a school at which any of the foregoing can be taught because the teaching develops with the emergence of a service such as healing. From service rendered gifts are grown. Knowledge increases; great increase of power follows and in the flowering of such power in time mankind must meet its needs.

The progressive nature of the spirit-directed mission to uncover truths long suppressed is shown by this incident in Edwards' development. We have seen how he moved from the recording of individual healings and the gathering of records to the just-concluded statement of a remarkable advance in technique, dependent upon a form of conscious co-operation with spirit doctors.

We have seen that concentration tends to defeat its purpose by creating tension as though each situation demanded, at least, great exertion. In the West we equate action with movement and achievement not realising that the mind is king and that will needs neither muscle nor increased blood pressure. In the West our passion is spent to win and, unfortunately, at all costs, usually meaning abuse of such spiritual gifts as surrender to the inner nature. Some of us sing the hymn, "Praise God From Whom All Blessings Flow" (as though God requires praise) then immediately we thwart the blessings by their abuse. In such a psychology of physical movement as the criterion of success it is supremely difficult for the spirit to express itself by becoming as the light of dawn, silent and serene. How do we "survive", or even prosper as we do? But, do we indeed prosper, or are our lives all spent, century by century, in attempts to right old wrongs and new misdeeds accumulate? Can the silent, inward way serve our needs in matters spiritual? Let us together now see.

Much is said about healing by thought. The saying and doing is not by Spiritualists alone. Many groups do so, mostly in a manner either unaware of the spirit or resistant to the claim that indeed even those who oppose Survival as a fact must themselves survive and witness how much they lose by not seeking to prove what they so strongly assert.

Meditation is an excellent exercise; so is concentration. Neither is required in healing at a distance. It was, for many years in my experience, taught and practised that at a given time each day those for whom and by whom healing was requested, should concentrate or focus their minds and wills upon co-operation with the healer. Fact and experience shows this is not so; quite the reverse.

Edwards had for many years set timed appointments with patients at a distance upon the ground that their combined "forces" would achieve healing. A disaster changed his thinking; perhaps that is one purpose of disaster. In June, 1944, two German V-1 bombs destroyed his home. In the upheaval following he missed many appointments for absent healing. You would expect that since, apparently, the absent healing by appointment was increasingly successful, any break in the arrangement would, at least, reduce the effectiveness of healing. The opposite was demonstrated; concentration at a given time was not only not required; it was a hindrance since it produced tensions that inhibited the efforts of the spirit healers. Edwards found that patients made greater progress during unscheduled healings than under the former set time arrangement.

The calm mind and the stilled emotions, the best

conditions for healing, especially absent healing, are difficult for a sick person to achieve. To require scheduled concentration in a person afraid, in pain or otherwise distressed is asking more than most can achieve. We humans expect results upon demand, on request, because we live such structured lives and are under such pressures that we rarely are still in mind and emotion although we may be at rest to all appearances.

We have witnessed the intensity of some praying, especially among evangelistic groups where the Deity is alternately harangued and implored and the praying cleric works hard to generate an atmosphere of emotion and excitement supposedly an aid to healing. In my native Britain this is not much seen but in my adopted country emotionalism and enthusiasm are consciously, deliberately stimulated under the mistaken belief that noise and excitement will somehow generate an unnamed power sufficiently to heal what is neither diagnosed nor understood. From personal inquiry I have confirmed that the efforts of some powerful psychics, working unknowingly with spirit healers, do achieve remarkable healings in public in spite of the atmosphere generated.

I am also aware from experience that in the United States healing by evangelists is inhibited by the resistant force of fixed doctrinal views. In Britain the religious atmosphere, especially in Spiritualism, is free from creedal rigidity and abuse of emotion. The superior nature and number of healings automatically follows.

Edwards again changed his procedure following cancellation of fixed time appointments by beginning his co-operation with his healing guides only after the long day's work was done, mostly after midnight when most patients would be asleep. Patients are expected to make weekly reports. As they progress or change he bears in mind that the healing be directed to specific conditions as well as to the general condition for which healing was sought originally. In this way, over the years, he has learned much of the nature of healing and of the process of recovery. By close association with his spirit sources he is enabled to tell patients what will be the next stage of recovery. All letters on healing are answered personally. The organisation is efficient; the stream of requests for healings goes on and on.

I wrote in April, 1948, that at the Shere sanctuary letters were received at the rate of 3,500 weekly. Since then it increased to more than 10,000 until the 15 million mark has been passed. You can anticipate the scepticism of those who are ignorant of the facts when such numbers are stated. From November, 1944, recoveries increased from 33 percent to 50 percent, and according to the disease, to between 85 and 90 percent.

Earlier it was stated that from many years' experience Edwards distilled statements of the operation of the healing forces and of his methods of co-operation. In his daily, silent communication with the spirit healers he has developed a gift of becoming aware of a patient's condition to such a degree that when patients reply to his letter in response to the first appeal for help, they report that he has gone to the roots of their troubles. In his communication or communion he is guided as to the course healing will follow until there is a cure or until there is a substantial improvement. It is from many years of such experiences that he has shaped a concept of the natural laws involved.

One of these laws is that there is a direct connection between the patient's mental state in such illness as epilepsy, rheumatism, heart, stomach and skin diseases. Taking skin disease as an example, he says that in every instance the patient reporting mentioned mental stress. The healer's first act is to calm the patient's mind. That result achieved, blood condition improves, the body acquires better tone, angriness of the skin surface or sores diminishes, the area of dead, scaly skin decreases. New skin covers the patches and the patient's outlook is brightened.

This is how the healer states the situation: ". . . in watching the weekly progress of healing invariably it is found that healing is in two phases. In the first there is general body betterment, as shown by more vitality, sounder sleep, and an inward uplift producing a happier, brighter outlook. Almost every patient writes to tell of this in the first week, and it is progressively maintained until they feel very fit. The second phase then commences, during which is seen the removal of the primary cause of the suffering and consequent lessening and removal of pain, stiffness, etc. It has frequently been noted that the effects of phases one and two are seen together, according to the nature of the illness."

It is a source of satisfaction as I recall reporting in *Psychic News*, in December, 1944, the first five cases of healing in which, Edwards said, the patients did not know of the treatment as it was being given. The facts remain as originally stated. Since I am persuaded there is no story so absorbing as the human story, you will understand why the following is a reproduction of what occurred so many years ago. The newspaper account I wrote 30 years ago has not been challenged in any particular. Here are selections from that revealing story:

"These healings cannot be the result of faith or the exercise of the patient's determination to get well by the exercise of will power. They are testimony to the reality of the law of human survival. They could only have been achieved through the control and administration of natural healing forces unknown to man, by discarnate minds which have progressed in knowledge of healing.

"The first case was of a woman who wrote on behalf of a friend, out of sympathy with Spiritualism. She was suffering from cancer of the breast. She was, wrote the friend, very ill . . . and the doctor at the hospital gave no hope of a cure and seemed to be resigned to that.

"The patient already had one breast removed and was receiving radium treatment on the other. Edwards began treatment on September 19, and a week later this letter was received: 'You will rejoice with me, I know, when I tell you she (the patient) started work last Monday after being home many weeks. Her only trouble seems to be a terrible soreness under her arm where radium has been used . . . There has been a return of appetite, no sickness whatever, whereas before her food was returned soon after eating . . . The return to health is going to be placed to the hospital's credit, but you and I are not going to worry about that'.

"Treatment was continued. The healer asked for information about the painful condition under the arm, which was very wet. The healer's experience is that cancers are sometimes discharged from the body in perspiration.

"On October 4 this letter was received: 'Miss ——— (the patient) is feeling very well in herself. The under-arm soreness and wetness have gone and new flesh is beginning to grow . . . I think that the moistures must have started round about the time you first began to treat her. Miss ——— has given up visiting the hospital now.' "

Then there was the case of the young man who sought healing for his fiancée, suffering since childhood from the distressing disease psoriasis. He wrote: "The doctor has been using a new remedy but it is having no result at all . . . She is feeling terribly distressed . . . She has had this complaint all her life . . . it has never been as bad as it is now . . . We hope to be married soon."

Fifteen days later the young man wrote: "I cannot begin to tell you how much happiness you have brought us . . . The improvement is wonderful. She can't believe her skin is really clearing up after this long time. When I wrote you, most of her body was covered with an angry redness . . . it was so bad that her nerves were seriously affected. Since writing to you the change has been nothing short of miraculous . . . There is no sign now of the dried flakes of skin that used to fall to the floor like confetti . . . She has this trouble from childhood and had many doctors, but they have never been able to cure her, so you can imagine how happy she is now."

Another case selected from the five in that one category is of a woman who for a year was in a mental institution. In accepting her for treatment Edwards said she would soon be home on parole. At that time I wrote:

"Eleven days later a letter was received from someone who had sought healing for the mental patient: 'She certainly seemed a little brighter . . . The doctor has granted us permission to have her home Saturday and Sunday.' "

The next report, a week later, said: "I am very pleased to tell you that when ——— was home last week-end she was decidely much better. She was much quicker in her actions, indeed, seemed much brighter and happier altogether."

This comment was added in the newspaper report: "In the cases cited the period of healing necessary for results was from one to three weeks, and in all of them appreciable recovery was made from the first day of treatment. All letters dealing with these cases have been checked."

Consider the three cases quoted out of five:

One woman, with breast cancer, was at least indifferent to Spiritualism; one was a mental patient; one had a serious skin disease from birth. If faith could have cured surely these cases provided prime opportunities for a demonstration of such a claim.

So much experience has accumulated in spirit healing that if faith were a decisive or even a contributing factor, it would not negate one iota of the claims made.

That is no reason for deriding faith, the very concept of which is comforting to many who have not thought through the implications of the claims on that head as fostered by believers in orthodox religion. It is wrong to claim that faith, of itself, which is a form of foretelling through hope, has no value. The approach should be that we strive to realise what we hope is true and desirable and beneficial and that by holding such thoughts in our minds maybe we will be strengthened in our resolves.

But, when we are faced with the questions raised by the situations just recounted, we should frankly ask ourselves: Why did not faith, any faith, achieve the same kind of results as the spirit physicians achieved through Edwards? Is he a repository of a special kind of faith? No, but he is an instrument for a special kind of healing.

It is no part of the aim of this story to destroy the faith of any soul; it is the aim to tell the truth as it is demonstrated and that we leave no question unexplored in our search. Faith, then, is not the explanation of the cause of success of spirit healing which, as so often stated, is achieved by the application of energies through knowledge to specific physical, mental, emotional and spiritual problems.

Leaving aside questions of faith, let us look at cases of cures that defy all criticism. There is little point now in presenting statistics, tabulating diseases or disorders, since we are in a situation running into some 15,000,000 applications for healing. The figure should be staggering in newspaper language.

Why should we be staggered? Only because sickness and disease are so menacing to most of us that the prospect of such healing causes, first, confusion then disbelief, then consideration and when experienced directly or through someone we know, causes a change of mind. I do not feel aggrieved when someone either scoffs at spirit healing or seeks an alternative explanation. The immensity of the change of thought wrought by the few cases stated even here must shock those who have no foreknowledge of even the probability of such healing. But, when the most illustrative of cases are reported, we have to concede that such success is sensational. And when it involves 15,000,000 people over 45 years it far exceeds anything of the kind reported as fact in holy books or wrought into fables.

There is no room left for alternative views as to cause. To paraphrase and slightly alter a quotation from Goldsmith's "Deserted Village", and substituting Edwards for the characters referred to: "They gazed and gazed and still the wonder grew that one small man could so much wonder do". The poet was referring to the village schoolmaster. I am referring to one man, with a limited formal education, without medical or scientific degrees, who, raised up by the spirit, has exceeded the healing achievements of all historical figures to whom many pray for relief of suffering. Their works are embellished because in the time they were done there were no analyses, no critical surveys, no checks of cures, little authentication since questions of creedal faith were involved—and nothing was taken away through the passing years. So are myths and legends made. So are new thoughts stifled.

But here, still before us, is the man and his colleagues who by loyalty to their teachers and guides in the spirit have changed thought, which most surely is an achievement equalled by few. The healer and his associates are here and now and may be seen, spoken to and estimated. They are not aloof, do not have titles, may be touched and heard and witnessed as they go about the business of life—healing and teaching; healing distress now, teaching of the better day that is coming because nothing otherwise will satisfy the press and urgent drive of life itself. We are indeed fortunate to live in such a time as this, for while in ages past our predecessors dreamed of deliverance from many ills, we have it so here, now and in abundance. And as these women and men have done and are doing, we may do so likewise. Is not this an exciting time?

Since it is tedious to write a story about statistics, let us look at some instances. We may choose to begin with either: "Once upon a time" or with: "There was a man, or woman". Better, let us begin with: "Once upon a time there was a disease. Not a tale of kings and queens and heroes and villains of battles won and lost but of healing."

A medium telephoned Edwards seeking aid for an alcoholic whose wife had left him. Within two weeks of the first absent healing the man changed his conduct. His wife returned to him. A check after three months showed the couple were still together. The husband's drinking problem had not returned. Many drink addicts have sought healing. The percentage of recoveries is high.

There is no known limit to the kind of cases relieved or cured by spirit healing. A woman in her twenties suffered a spinal displacement in an accident. She had manipulative treatment from osteopaths and doctors. A childbirth strain aggravated her condition. Edwards and a few associates gave healing as she lay on a couch. Her mother helped in the healing. Edwards entranced the patient. Treatment then began. This report was made by the mother:

"In a very short while, actually only a matter of seconds, the healer's hands appeared to grasp the backbone on either side of the displacement. The backbone appeared to be lifted upwards under the skin, the sections of the bone put into line and the backbone replaced. As a considerable time has now elapsed since my daughter had the operation on her back, it is possible to judge the results.

"Her trouble dated from a motor accident some fifteen years ago and she has suffered considerable pain in her back ever since although she has had osteopathic treatment, massage, etc. The operation performed by Mr. Harry Edwards cured her of this longstanding pain, and I feel I must send you a line with my sincere thanks and warm appreciation. I want to thank you for the permission of allowing me to witness the miracle, for I could never have believed unless I had seen with my own eyes how wonderful it was. Her spine was lifted quite three inches from its normal place. No human being could have done such a thing."

Since statistics do not live or speak, or feel, it is better we stay with people while the columns of figures stand sentinel over the achievements in spirit healing. Most of the people I know and with whom I talked while writing this book say they are impressed most by accounts of individual healings. This brings home to them the feeling that they might have to call upon such a healing as is told in this case:

"She was born a weakling and not expected to live. From her earliest days her life was one long series of illnesses. In adult years acute throat trouble was added to her burden. She underwent several operations, and in the years that followed she spent long intervals in bed. Then came spinal trouble, followed by painful internal ailments. There were regular medical experimental treatments and operations. Doctors took a very sympathetic interest in her case, but the medical records were marked 'incurable' and 'beyond recovery'."

"A friend of this patient wrote asking Edwards for absent healing. There was an immediate response for the better. Pain and loss of weight ceased and a general movement towards recovery began. From the time spirit healing was requested she did not have any surgical or medical treatment other than a tonic medicine. This woman said she felt her body being worked upon by 'invisible hands'. Her health continued to improve to such an extent that she found work in government service."

That account is summarised from a newspaper report but is typical of the Edwards file of the most complex cases. I wrote many years ago that in research of such files it was difficult to decide when to stop. Only the unique, rare cases, and a few other categories are filed. No private individual could afford to maintain a file that has long passed the 15 million mark.

I surmise that when an article written by me for *Psychic News* of the healing mission of Kathryn Kuhlman, an American evangelist, a few British eyebrows might have been raised because of the uninhibited show preceding the healing. That is why it was and is news. It is news because she has been loyal to her spirit mentors, whereas the male American evangelists who are healers have moved on to the greener pastures where money appears to grow on trees, all to be had for the picking. I know these men can heal and they are proud of it, but their interest is elsewhere. Kuhlman, nearing 70, is at work always carrying a schedule of meetings few men could equal. And she heals in public, which for the sceptical must be a challenge. That is why I saw her at work. If there were 50 or even five, or even one, male equivalent in America much could be done for the nation. Britain, in that respect, is more fortunate in its healers.

Healing has been a public question for a long time

because sickness has been a public matter for a long time. I had seen several others at work, and in my own ignorance of the facts had tried to heal others, I hope out of compassion. Good intentions may justify inadequate performance. So when reporting my first experience of Edwards at work in public, this is what happened.

The Kingsway Hall, London, was filled to capacity. Many healers were present, by arrangement, to co-operate. A girl is brought up to the platform. A hand, paralysed. Edwards dealt with her spine. In a few moments she cried out, "I am cured". No manipulation, just the almost caressing touch of the healer's hand. Simple, speedy—a cure of paralysis brought on by shock caused when, in her bath, she heard an air raid siren moaning its warning. Here is what I wrote then:

"As she sat in the chair, Edwards spoke to her, as he did to all of them to distract their attention from the healing. He turned her so that her back was to the audience and with his finger traced the curvature of the spine. A doctor who was invited to the platform to see what was happening also observed the degree of curvature from the normal. The doctor was a stranger to the healer. He agreed with all the statements made by Edwards about the spines of patients whom he treated, except in one case where he said he could not tell what happened because of the patient's clothing.

"Without using force, which he says is unnecessary in healing, Edwards placed his fingers across the backbone and shortly afterwards said simply, 'That's beautiful, that's done'. Then he showed the audience how stiff the girl's elbow was. He moved it gently, and slowly took it up higher and higher until the girl was touching the back of her head. It was then he asked how long it was since she had done that, but she said quietly, her face covered with a smile of wonder, 'I am cured'. Her fingers had before bent upwards, but now they were moving at her desire as she looked at them. The paralysed arm made whole."

Edwards worked for more than an hour, healing 12 persons. He stopped because he felt a tension in the huge hall. He is a pioneer of the need for the relaxed approach in healing, since he knows by experience how tension defeats what the sick most desire, hence his emphasis on absent healing where there is, in the night, no tension—only the silent spirit healers at their benign service free from the emotion and thoughts of many who have been sick and suffering for years.

In contrast, the American healer Kuhlman deliberately stimulates her audiences. When a peak of tension is developed the healing begins, almost in a stream of patients to the platform.

The very thought that healing might come to one of them first brings up the feelings of the audience. I have observed that phenomenon elsewhere, especially in evangelistic gatherings where the emotions are deliberately stimulated in the ill-informed expectation that somehow, in a manner unexplained since it is not understood, a spiritual power, of which the preachers and undeveloped healers have no knowledge, will manifest itself without knowledge—and that a spectacular cure will result.

I do not write that in any spirit of carping or of superiority, but the fact is that relatively few healings are seen in such an atmosphere while the expectations continue—a mixture of religion, superstition and fear—fear that healing will not come. I do not expect all who live by their creeds and superstitions to shed them because I, or anyone else, shows that there is a better way—the way of knowledge in healing by the spirit through healers who know what is being done in the cause of health—and knowledge.

So, we resume the story. Before Edwards decided that tension was developing, he had brought relief to a deaf woman, telling her that much of her trouble was due to her straining to catch sounds.

Another woman, deaf in both ears, improved so much that the healer tested the effect by walking slowly away from the patient who had her back turned to him. She said she heard his voice, unchanging in volume, up to a distance of six feet.

The deaf are made to hear.

The healer asked that only those cases said by doctors to be incurable be brought to him. The first was of a man with a deformed foot. The doctor had mounted the platform in response to Edwards' call and tested the man's statement that he could not move the affected foot sideways. He said he had received medical aid for nine years. Before a hushed audience Edwards touched the foot and easily it moved sideways, making a creaking sound. When asked, the man said he did not feel pain. I sat a few feet from the point on the platform where healing was given, watching the faces for signs of the pain usual in cases of medical manipulation.

Edwards does not manipulate. He does encourage movement, for reasons already stated—the limb or area treated has its own consciousness which responds to healing. I have seen—and experienced—osteopathic manipulation and have felt pain, followed by relief. In the case of the man with the deformed foot, it seemed to co-operate as Edwards spoke to it, turning it slowly until it was supple. The man wiggled his toes, which he said he had not been able to do for years.

And the lame were made to walk.

Next came a woman with a set spine. The doctor confirmed her statement. Edwards knelt before the woman, and said as he placed her arms on his shoulders, that she had endured her set spine for 10 years and that two and a half years before seeing Edwards was told her case had "exhausted medical knowledge".

As they swayed together, a strange sight on that Saturday afternoon in a large, hushed hall, the healer said, "Let your backbone yield". The doctor placed a hand on the woman's spine as the healer, still swaying with the woman, said: "There is no human knowledge that can remove that condition", meaning that the healing was being done by spirit power.

Then he caused the woman to bend slowly, gently backwards. Soon she leaned backwards of her own accord. Again the spine. Edwards now healed her leg, affected by the spinal condition. The patient showed she could walk more freely. She had come to the platform, stiffly. Then she looked as though her spine was fixed but now, following the healing, she walked with a supple movement. And how happy she looked.

Next came a woman who, for 28 years, suffered a condition of the spine so far advanced and displaced that it showed under one shoulder blade. Edwards informed the audience that he had given this woman healing before but could not remedy the whole defect there and then because the ribs were also displaced. Even in face of that, the doctor, who watched as the treatment was being given, agreed that the spine had been straightened for some distance. The patient volunteered the statement that she had been much helped by the one treatment just given.

Then there was the instance of the woman who had to be taken away for removal of her spinal jacket before Edwards could treat her. She received attention later.

In her place came another woman, so paralysed she dragged one leg. She handed a note to Edwards saying her speech was affected by the paralysis which spread down her right side.

She had two curvatures of the spine.

Edwards asked the doctor to place his hands on the spine, saying to him: "I want you to feel the movement as it takes place". As he said so, gently he moved the body. The doctor said the spine straightened. To this day, after so many years, I can almost hear the hush in that hall. I looked quickly at the audience. It was like a painting by an artist of a bygone age representing, A Case of Healing.

Edwards then said he had removed the pressure on the woman's nerves and had asked his spirit guides to restore the affected hand. The patient was asked to grip the handrail at the edge of the platform to show the audience that her grip had been restored. The leg which she could not stand on before was treated next. Soon she was rising on her toes.

Edwards urged those in the audience who for years had suffered through loss of the use of a limb to seek healing at Spiritualist churches. Healing, he declared, is one power for the service of all who suffer and it was a mighty power. He did not claim a monopoly. Many others could also heal.

A boy wearing an iron brace over a wasted leg was urged to walk after treatment. He did so, He had been paralysed from the age of three. He, so lately started, would have to learn to walk afresh. But he did look confident as he held the healer's hand and took a few steps along the platform.

It made no difference on that memorable day which kind of problem was placed before the healer. A woman who suffered from rheumatoid arthritis lifted a stiffened leg, swung it awkwardly at first, then freely. She began a walk with Edwards, at her suggestion. On their way down the steps from the platform the healer stopped to treat her stiffened elbow. Then together, holding hands, they completed their walk.

You might here ask: Where was official medicine in

all of this? I could not, for his sake, give the young doctor's name. But all opposition would have been helpless in face of the living facts—the healing of many by spirit power who had nowhere to go but to the spirit.

And they each went their several ways, each to their homes, and there was much rejoicing as the news was carried abroad of many who had suffered and were now whole.

Then to the climax. There now came forward a man, leaning on a stick. For 20 years his burden had been disseminated sclerosis, his back stiff as a rod. He could not bend. In less than one minute following a treatment he bent, touched his toes, first standing then sitting. Edwards was not satisfied so he treated the leg which had been stiff for 20 years. The man who had shuffled up to the platform now walked across it with Edwards, still with the aid of his stick but no longer shuffling. The healer told the man that after 20 years of restriction the legs would require time to return to their normal function.

Several times there was applause which probably eased the tension which caused Edwards to halt at 12 cases healed—each striking, and each of such a character that no doctor would publicly treat such cases.

There were 50 other healers on the platform on that day of healing. It is certain their gifts were merged to support what the spirit healers were doing. Edwards has always urged those who require further healing to go to other healers who would complete the treatment. Some healers say they do not care to "mix" the power. Since that is not under their control, the claim does not appear to have much to recommend it. Perhaps personal considerations prevail. However that may be, Edwards always recommends the simplest, most natural, relaxed approach. The healing is all, let it be done, and all is well.

The Healer of Shere's healing in that Kingsway Hall demonstration is only one of hundreds of such achievements throughout his 45 years of service. He says little of the healers in the spirit who are the heart, mind and skill of the mission. On one occasion a clairvoyant saw two famous predecessors of Edwards, Billy Parish and Fred Jones, renowned in their time for the total and variety of healings. These two were seen at Edwards' side, which is the way it should be.

Of the spirits who are the directors of the mission I know little. Lister, a famous British doctor in his day, is one. Pasteur, noted French scientist, is another.

Edwards, as already reported, tells of his development, his gift of trance speaking and so on. Few outside the centre of Spiritualism know that mediumship is not a college syllabus art: it is a result of development of a gift or gifts brought to earth by the aspiring soul. When the time is ripe, the spirit people who are to co-operate with the potential instrument make their impressions on the mind. Life begins to change as test upon test is met. There arrives a day on which the realisation comes of the dawning of mediumship. Some instruments reach a plateau and continue their work from it. Others, according to their natures and desires, exhibit new aspects; some are able to co-operate consciously with their guides, a condition which many of them prefer since it achieves what has been planned. This is not the place for a full analysis of mediumship which is beyond any person in the flesh since we see only in small part what is a significant and complex whole. But it is the basis of genius—the forerunner of the distant time when what is genius now will be the norm then.

Our Healer of Shere has learned by experience and choice to work consciously at various levels of expression without requiring to be entranced. He has achieved what is most desired—the blending of consciousness in which much may be achieved since the medium becomes a more receptive, supple and expressive instrument. His goal is healing: whatever impedes that being achieved is laid aside. There are other mediums highly capable of serving other ends.

My personal experience with Edwards is all at what is called the normal level, if we can discover what is normal. But I do recall an experience when gathering material for the book, *Born to Heal.* Harry asked me to sit in a large, high-backed chair. I did so. We talked about the research material. I began to stammer. Those who know me well know I do not stammer. Quite the reverse. Edwards laughed at my predicament in efforts to correct the stammer. He told me the influence was of a spirit guide who, on earth, stammered. A test? No. A demonstration of mind influencing mind, yes. Maybe that says more than many words—and theories.

It is easy to understand the reaction of many to such reports as are given here and elsewhere of feelings such as described. What is the force that straightens a spine, cures arthritis of long standing? Let us look at some instances then try to find explanations.

A spine is rigid, has been so for many years. The healer lightly moves a hand from the neck to the bottom of the spine which straightens up and becomes flexible as you watch. There is no phsyical force involved. What is required to be done is done by a power transmitted through Edwards (or other healers) of such nature that the condition called poker back is cured, and the sufferer is free from pain and handicap. You may choose to deny one case of a claimed cure of such an ailment. Then one case becomes two, these become three, and they multiply until the score is by the thousands, few by comparison with the total by physical contact. Most cures are by distant or absent healing. I am aware that it seems too good to be true. It is true that by the tens and hundreds of thousands they are healed. An intelligence superior to the healer's applies energy or energies to affected limbs and so changes the chemical condition which produces the poker back state that natural movement is recovered —the "incurable" is cured.

If that, basically, is not so, then we have a situation beyond reason, nature, art, science and commonsense.

You have read of a doctor taking part in a public demonstration of healing of locked limbs. That was in London in clear view of a large audience. Here is a case of like healings at Redhill, Surrey, where members of the St. John Ambulance Brigade brought sufferers to the biggest hall in town where Edwards was healing. He selected the chronic cases, the incurables, including various aspects of paralysis, disseminated sclerosis, arthritis, locked limbs and spinal curvatures.

The captain of the ambulance brigade unit was invited to the platform to witness the treatment. This is what happened:

Edwards asked the captain to place her fingers on one side of each vertebra while he touched the opposite side. The healing began. The vertebrae separated. The spine was freed from its rigid position. The captain readily confirmed the movement. She now became a test witness: She was asked to place her hands in the small of the patient's back, the medium moving away, asking the patient to arch her back by herself. This she did. Again the ambulance brigade captain said the spine was flexible.

There followed similar co-operation in a case of double spinal curvature: one curve outward, the other sideways. With the captain's fingers interlocked with his, the healer gently moved the patient's body until the spine was straight.

Only three cases failed to show immediate response. Patients who had been helped up the steps to reach the platform descended by themselves, with the exception of a blind woman. Those who used canes for support returned to their seats without these aids.

One of the spinal cures of that evening, if achieved in a hospital or an orthodox church, would have been hailed as a miracle. With Edwards, then, and in the ensuing years it had become almost commonplace. But to the person healed there is no such state as commplace: To each one it is outstanding.

Edwards has healed in most areas of Britain and has visited other countries. The striking cases abound. Here is one that must move even the most sceptical; it occurred in the crowded Newcastle upon Tyne City Hall. A young mother gazed intently as Harry passed his hand over the head of Margaret Ritchie, aged four, of North Shields, stone deaf since she was one year old. Margaret stared at the healer's face as he treated her. The healer clicked his finger nails. The child responded. Edwards said: "She is healed now".

The mother, in the body of the hall, cried out: "That's my bairn", and fainted.

A girl with a spinal deformity was a piteous sight—the backbone was behind a shoulder blade. Her knees were locked. She could not walk. The spine, under Edwards' healing, responded and slowly moved from behind the shoulder blade. Edwards said: "As the spine is now clear the shoulder blade should go back into its correct position". He placed a hand on the shoulder. The audience gasped as it was seen that the deformity had gone.

The knees did not yield so readily. But as Edwards treated them the spine had further straightened until it was almost centered on the back. And this occurred without Edwards' contact because he was then treating the knees.

To study reports of this healing in order to select

prime examples is like walking through a vast plain of roses, all in full bloom where you decide "now", then glimpsing another more beautiful. There is no end. Yet some choices must be made to present, at least, a picture of what in another age would have been hailed as "miracles".

Could simple faith, psychological reaction, expectation or any other theory explain the following?:

A woman wrote Edwards: "I had another medical examination and the surgeon was pleased to see there is a vast difference. He was astonished at the change of position of the womb, and stated that from being upside down it is now completely normal."

If the change resulted from psychological reaction why did not the surgeon cause that condition?

Another: "The doctor says the impossible has happened, and the operation will not be necessary".

The instances just given were selected from 100 cases in the first four months of one year, all concerning removal of diseased areas or changes in diseased organs to such an extent that operations projected by surgeons were avoided. These surgeons so decided upon the basis of changed conditions with which they had nothing to do.

It is a logical question: How do doctors feel about spirit healing? That depends upon the individual doctor since we cannot take all medical women and men as mere statistics. It was difficult for most doctors, trained in an orthodoxy based upon some scientific principles, to admit into their minds the concept of energies beyond energy as they understand it and upon the action of entities said to be our own kind translated to another world or consciousness by the mere, natural act of dying.

Because this section reports, and comments, upon doctors—and their families—being healed where all else failed, they remain anonymous. The reason is plain:

they, if they stated their successful appeals for spirit healing, would be deprived of their livelihoods—a strange threat, but, to most, persuasive.

Early in his healing mission Edwards was asked by a woman doctor living in the country to give healing to a member of her medical staff. The doctor had been so advised by a spirit who spoke to her at a seance. By absent healing the staff member recovered, regaining lost weight and vigour. Then the doctor sought healing for herself. She wrote that she was unwell, losing weight and feeling "like nothing else on earth . . . I lost two stone in two months and could hardly crawl about". It was difficult for her to walk upstairs to consultations at patients' homes. A doctor she saw professionally said she was suffering from anxiety leading to heart attacks. He did not state a basic cause of his medical colleague's troubles.

The ailing doctor asked Edwards for distant healing; she did not give details of her case or condition. The result was: "On Christmas morning," she wrote, "I suddenly felt better and had a big dinner for the first time in ages. From that moment I have felt a different being and have put on weight at the rate of one pound a week. I no longer get heart attacks, and at this rate I shall soon be normal again."

The recovered doctor who had been advised by an unseen spirit at a seance to seek Edwards' aid when her own doctor had failed, then added: "I dare not write an account for publication. It would be an unpardonable sin from the medical point of view. Though I do not care what people think, I dare not risk getting crossed off the register and so lose my livelihood."

But—when some doctors, in their ignorance of the realities of the benefits of spirit healing, attack it they are not anonymous. They are taking advantage of a privileged position while ready to impose sanctions on others—not only for the sake of an opinion but for the maintenance of power. Dare we say that preservation of income is also a strong motive? Yes, I do.

At that point in the healing saga the medical profession, as represented by the British Medical Association, had not been compelled by its self-interest to attack spirit healing. The initial reaction was one of disdain, somewhat lofty, but still disdain which was eroded, healing by healing, of doctors and their families, all acknowledged anonymously, for reasons just given. Official medicine had to try to discredit healing: it was too successful.

In a letter to Edwards, a doctor in the South of England wrote:

"You will, I hope, remember that after your remarkable demonstration of spiritual healing at ———— last Sunday I had the pleasure of shaking hands with you. You may recollect that at the time I was very distressed because my mother had that day had a fall and a stroke and was lying unconscious without the slightest hope of recovery.

"You promised me that you would put her on your healing list. It is with a feeling of deep gratitude to God, to yourself and to your co-workers in spirit that I write to say that my mother has not only recovered consciousness, but the speech centre which for days was paralysed—she was unable to articulate a word—has suddenly functioned again. She is talking almost normally and is taking a bright and intelligent interest in all that goes on around her.

"Her own doctor gave very little hope of her recovering her speech again, and in over 30 years of medical practice I have not known such a miraculous recovery. My mother will be 87 if she lives to September 15 next. This speaks for itself."

That is not the end of that doctor's debt to spirit

healing. His letter requests absent healing be given to his daughter, suffering from pulmonary tuberculosis and to his sister, who had osteo-arthritis, adding:

"It would give me great pleasure to meet you again, and I will let no professional engagements, other than the most vital, stand in the way if you will give me the opportunity."

A postscript states: "My sister has just told me that the doctor in attendance has expressed himself as being amazed, and that he never expected my mother to recover."

This doctor is a casebook. He lists the following healings:

"With my warmest thanks for your treatment of my neck. There is slight but definite improvement in my neck and eyes. It would be, I think, unreasonable to expect any more considering the number of years I have been suffering from both."

Then he reports on several persons for whom he sought healing:

"Mrs. B., aged 77, curvature (of the spine) and heart. Curvature less marked. Pain is not so frequent and she can sit up straighter, i.e., without so much stoop.

Another Mrs. B.: "Painful knee of one year's standing. No pain in the knee since receiving your treatment. Cure apparently complete.

"My brother, feared commencing arthritis in the hip. Very slight pain now. Much improved.

"My sister, aged 58, osteo-arthritis in right hip of four and a half years' standing and valvular disease of the heart. Regret to report no change but she only had two treatments.

"My wife, for over four years was unable to lie in bed after awakening without in a few minutes being assailed with a headache so severe that she was hardly able to move. A blinding headache would best describe it.

About two months ago you felt down my wife's cervical spine and remarked, 'Ah, here's your trouble' and rested your fingers for a moment on one of the vertebrae—it would be interesting to know which. My wife says you did not manipulate the spine in any way. This was her first and last treatment, for since then she has had no sign of headache.

"I cannot ascribe the cure to anything but spiritual healing, for my wife is not a Spiritualist and up to this experience had no faith in anything of the kind. She was, in fact, rather inclined to pooh-pooh the whole thing, and at the same time no one was more surprised than myself when she stepped forward to sit on your stool in front of you. Congratulations and warmest thanks."

The file of doctors seeking healing for themselves, families, friends—and patients—is revealing. There is no argument, no derogation, no air of superiority—only concerned souls seeking help wherever it may be found. The list is long and soon becomes repetitive. But, we all yield to temptation because it is so attractive. One instance that compels publication is of a doctor's wife seeking treatment for a middle-aged woman friend who had one operation for cancer. The surgeon prescribed deep x-ray therapy but said it could be only palliative. He thought the cancer would recur within a few months.

The doctor's wife who sought help for her friend had seen Edwards heal at a public meeting. She wrote: "My husband and I believe that spiritual healing can—if it is God's will—do what science does not yet know of. Will you help her, please?"

Another doctor's wife who sought healing for another person stated: "Miss ——— is now rapidly recovering from the severe reaction to the deep ray therapy and is able to get up each day and take normal diet."

Before reporting another side to some doctors' views

of spirit healing and spirit healers, it should be told that many cases of mental sickness have been healed without resort to electrical shock treatments. Frequently these illnesses are caused by the after-death interference of those who died unready, social problems, sick, angry or bound to earth by frustrated desires. These poor, unhappy souls are amenable to kindly persuasion. This I know from experience, as do many others. There is no great mystery here. But what certain churches and some foolish priests and ignorant thrill-seekers say and do is another matter.

Once released from their self-made attachment to a receptive victim, the invading entities resume their lives in the spirit. Cures of such cases excite little interest among Spiritualists because they know the causes and know also that a remedy is available.

Again, temptation defeats resolve because spirit healing has recorded successes with retarded children to the joy of parents who had tried orthodox treatments.

A woman was in danger of becoming obsessed through her own folly. An ignorant entity had become attached to her, causing much distress. Edwards responded to the call for healing from the husband who stated he was desperate. His wife was terrified that in the night the entity would try to control her. For some time she was bombarded day and night with efforts to control her. She was in deep distress when her husband wrote for absent healing. Three weeks later he wrote:

"I am more than grateful to know that the personality has been removed. My wife tells me that she is herself sure that it is with her no longer . . . I am glad to say that her nervous attacks are not as bad as they were." A week later he reported that "She is more or less entirely free from any disturbing influences now".

How is spirit surgery carried out? I do not know since the healers in the spirit do not tell. Questions of diagnosis arise. Doctors in this world have their problems even with sophisticated modern equipment. But diagnostic equipment of itself does not heal. Then there are errors in diagnosis, a situation which provides alibis for those doctors who deny spirit healing successes on the ground that the original diagnosis was in error. But the original diagnosis was made by a doctor, maybe even a specialist.

I expect that from the spirit position diagnosis goes more directly to the cause or causes than to the symptoms. What methods are used by spirit doctors I cannot say—but their healings are striking and their methods swift and their successes in most difficult cases, from our viewpoint, are sensational. They must know much more than we, or doctors, do because they achieve more and better, painlessly.

Although I have personal experience of spirit surgery it does not make me any wiser in the matter than someone who heard of it or experienced it only yesterday. There is no blood in psychic surgery, which is perhaps a misnomer since the body is not entered in the sense that a surgeon makes an incision. Since there is no severance of nerve or tissue, no surgery on bones, no loss of blood, generally no effect comparable to anaesthesia, how is the surgery done? Again, I do not know, but should it be discovered or disclosed before the word "finis" is written here, I will make a report. I have theories but they are too complex to be valid. There must be a simple explanation that covers the most ground.

Take this case, which I reported. An American soldier broke some ankle bones in a parachute jump, which kept him in hospital for eight weeks. Healing was slow. A friend gave him a copy of the *Psychic News* telling of a healer's success. The soldier was more than sceptical yet his friend urged him to ask for Edwards' help. He did so, then lost the healer's address.

A little later he danced at a farewell party, his ankle

hurt so he went to bed and slept. Abruptly he awakened, and by a light from a corridor, "saw a man arrayed in a white overall standing by his bed with his face turned away". He continues: "He seemed to put his hand right through the blankets, gripped my leg underneath the calf and brought the leg up through the blankets so that I could see it. He had a grip as strong as an iron wrench. With his other hand he grasped the foot and pulled it outwards away from the leg. Then with his fingers moved the bones in the ankle and let the foot go back. As he did this a great pain shot up my leg from the foot to the head. It was so paralysingly strong that I was helpless and could not even cry out. He placed my leg and foot again through the blanket, turned to me and smiled as if to say 'OK'. When he looked at me his face seemed to glow with a light much whiter than anything I have seen."

For a moment or two the soldier thought he was back in hospital and only after the figure disappeared did he see he was on his billet with the light on. He heard a comrade snore. He felt sure he was awake during the incident. To test the experience he got out of bed and examined his foot. Where it had been held there was a white band as if pressure had forced blood away from the area. In the morning the white band was faintly seen. He tried the healed foot. All stiffness had gone.

The soldier reported the incident to his doctor who did not appear surprised. Later he met the friend who had suggested he write to Edwards. The friend was speechless then recalled when he wrote to the healer . . . it was just two days before the healing incident. The friend received Edwards' reply on the day the healing occurred. The healer's letter was lost so the soldier asked *Psychic News* to tell Edwards what had occurred, and that he would write to him from his home in the U.S.A.

The young American's comment is: "All I know is

that after months of pain and stiffness the above did take place on the day the healer said it would be given. I am going home now. I have had a good time in your country and now I have something more to remember it by than any amount of dollars can buy."

That is a healing defiant of all theories of faith, spontaneity, human magnetism, healer's super-personality, persuasiveness, hypnotism, magnetism, pills, deep-ray therapy, psychiatry or psychology. If I have omitted any category it is only because of a limited vocabulary. I forgot—prayer, voodoo and shamanism were omitted.

One more and I have done because the record goes on and on. When you think "enough is enough" there comes another and yet another until you say stop. But wait. Several healings were investigated for Edwards by Mr. Leonard Shires, secretary at that time of the Leeds Psychic Research Society. Following a demonstration by Edwards of these this one is selected from among the healed persons and summarised, heavily.

George Proctor, of Normanton, Yorks., was born with a spinal curvature. He was nine years old before he walked, mainly by will power. He left his job in a foundry at 14—and collapsed. Fibrositis was the diagnosis. Treatment failed. Now osteo-arthritis and scoliosis was the diagnosis. He was hung by the neck while a plaster cast was applied. It had to be removed before setting. So, he was sent home until another cast could be applied. This he could not tolerate—off it came.

Yes, this is a summary of one man's woes. Another surgeon had Proctor placed in a metal frame only 10 inches wide, with chin and face straps. Head weights pulled at his neck apparently in an effort to straighten the spine.

The report goes on and on, plaster casts, hung up by the neck, and extra large cast. Still, he endured, a living mummy in a plaster sarcophagus—except that while he may not have been, in the ordinary sense, alive, he was breathing.

The surgeon in the case proposed three operations in six weeks to fuse the spine. Seven weeks Proctor passed in plaster. The surgeon released him from his plaster—and pain. He was at the end of his tether. It was suggested by the doctor that he visit a London spine specialist. In London, Proctor was told the Leeds surgeon wanted him back for surgery that would cure him. Surgery was done—spinal fusion.

For 18 weeks Proctor, anticipating a cure, lay on his back, cheerfully. Another spinal support was made Proctor got up. He could not endure more; the old pain had returned. Four weeks of psychiactric treatment followed. Some six weeks before Edwards visited Leeds, Proctor faced a disappointment—the healer had so many requests he could not be treated. He persevered. Edwards did treat him. Proctor felt at once that life for him was about to become better.

Proctor recovered sufficiently to follow the healer's advice to take on light work. He had, in his narrative, omitted one point: the initial healing had altered his back so much that his jacket had to be altered. Seven months later he wrote to Edwards that on his job he had to leave home at 6.30 a.m., walk a mile and a half after leaving the bus—and repeat the trip to get home, of course.

His comment is: "I feel very proud with Mr. Edwards and every one of you connected with him. I am ever so tired when I get home." Who would not be after his years of pain—and plaster and metal?

How does the healer feel, say, before a public demonstration? There is a view that you must be nervous or tense in speaking before an audience although no one has yet explained why this is supposed to be so. Since healing requires calm, Edwards is the calmest person in the hall before healing begins and remains so. He waits silently during the preliminaries, mentally notes those least able to stand and decides how he will heal them. There is no order of priority of those to be healed, as the preceding report and commentary shows. Since there are no priorities none can allege collusion for effect.

The healer states some limits to the effectiveness of healing: Where limbs are so weakened by disuse they cannot function, as in the case of legs incapable of supporting the body, or where by surgery bones have been removed—the body structure is so changed as to forbid the return of natural function.

The healer chooses the most difficult cases for demonstration. As they are brought forward he receives an inward diagnosis as to the cause and the point or points at which healing is to be applied. Say it is in a leg. He knows where the cause lies—in the limb, in the spine, or in a nerve centre in the brain. He is then aware only of the directional effort to deal with the cause. If that is in the spine, the now sensitive fingers are also aware. The diagnosis completed, the fingers sense the seat of trouble and the healing power flows. If the trouble is spinal curvature, the vertebrae are moved gently as you would move links in a chain. Then the vertebrae slide painlessly into place. Where the spinal condition is fixed, the fingers, with the gentle movement of the patient, achieve flexibility.

Physical force has no place in spirit healing. Edwards is positive no pain is caused. In his experience, pain has been caused only once. It was quickly removed and has not recurred. (Perhaps that occurred in the case of the American soldier, as described earlier.)

As soon as healing is accomplished the healer experiences happiness—because the work has been done.

The growth of intimate collaboration is the key to his

success. When his mission began he relied upon his faith because he could not fully realise he had succeeded.

When he knows the healing has been accomplished, then he can tell the patient to walk or stand up or do any other thing required to show what has been achieved. The healing itself is done in a flashing moment. He, in the face of many years of success, is still surprised by the speed of healing which sometimes occurs before he approaches the patient.

When all has been said about the healing, the huge totals of cases handled in a year, the complexity and longevity of many, there comes a time when so much experience may be distilled into a few precepts. Edwards expresses his experience in this statement of his foundation for doing what is done through him:

Supreme faith in the spirit doctors.
Avoid all personal techniques.
Healing is a simple act, as simple as a finger beckoning.
Appeal to, or attune with, the spirit realm rather than one spirit personality, and then know that all that can be done will be done.

Frequently I am asked, if spirit healing is true, why do the churches not adopt it; why don't doctors become healers, like Edwards and the thousands of healers claimed to be serving in Britain alone?

The answer is always that the road to becoming a healer/medium is open to all, on the same terms and under the same discipline.

Then, I am asked, what has to be done to become a healer? Is there a method which can be taught, a school at which instruction is given?

Then there are questions from those who reasonably maintain, as they should, faith in doctors and medical and surgical therapies and procedures.

Again, this is asked: have churches and medical

associations inquired into the claims made for healing? This is as appropriate a place as any to reply.

First, it is difficult for veterans in this work to have confidence in any body or group which conducts an inquiry then suppresses the favourable report resulting. An example is that of the Church of England's Commission on Spiritualism. The report was leaked to *Psychic News*. It showed that a majority of the Commission voted favourably.

There followed, after many years and a river of healings, a Church of England Commission on what it called divine healing. Edwards, invited to state a case, was coldly received. You may recall also the treatment he received from the medical committee of that commission. Doctors' support of healing was ignored. Edwards, as you also may recall, had a long experience of standing alone in advocating what he knows to be true of healing.

That church commission on "divine" healing, including its chosen doctors, heard from Edwards these compressed statements:

Restore the gift of healing to the church and it will become a living presence.

The gift of healing can never belong to the Church of England or to any other denomination. It is God's gift to all humanity.

There are no separate divine laws for each separate church; it is a common heritage.

Any attempt to monopolise healing will fail. Ritual, discipline, set prayers or the efforts of healing priests will fail.

Spiritual healing is divine in origin and purpose and is commanded by the founder of Christianity.

The terms divine healing and spiritual healing mean the same thing. Spirit healing comes from a non-human source. A healer is one who serves as an instrument of the non-human agency. No human being has in his own power the gift of healing.

Spirit healing cures the incurable—by medical definition. There is no limit to the range of healing. To cure the incurable requires power and knowledge beyond human achievement.

Healing rests on the truth of survival of bodily death which is one reason for church rejection since it is linked with Spiritualism.

In his peroration, Edwards declared: "I hold that the divine purpose behind the healing is not so much the healing of the sick but that through this healing the spiritual consciousness will be aroused. They see themselves and their dear ones healed by spiritual means. This provides a demonstration of spiritual power that is so sorely needed in this scientific age. Restore the gift of healing to the Church and it will become a vital and living presence. I need not tell you how great is the need for this in our world today."

Eloquent, moving—and true. The Church's response: Silence.

What evidence did Edwards offer that Church Commission? You will recall the incredible outburst by a doctor when offered files of 70 recent "incurables" who had been healed. Edwards did not say they were incurable. Doctors in the cases had done so. The Commission's doctor cried: "These are not proof of spiritual healing. The results could have been achieved by spontaneous or natural healing." To which Edwards replied that the doctor's statement was a monstrous evasion because the patients named had been described as incurable. Again the official evasion on which medical orthodoxy rests: "Too many doctors are describing cases as incurable."

There is, in medical terms, no cure for medical evasion. Not even truth will suffice.

That is intentional repetition to show how stubborn are otherwise reasonable men, when their cherished beliefs are threatened by knowledge new to them; it is a universal, continuing malady.

That is the reason behind the conduct of the Commission on Healing established by the Archbishops of Canterbury and York. Could Edwards the healer, with all of his accomplishments, receive a fair hearing? After all, these two powerful men, claiming by virtue of their office a special place in the world, were facing a challenge without precedent. A man, a Spiritualist, was bold enough to say, and even demonstrate, that he could heal where doctors failed. He also claimed he had proof and offered documents and cases to substantiate that proof. That could not be tolerated.

Edwards, a kindly man whose very gentleness is at the root of his receptivity to spirit power, was shocked by the treatment he received. He had hoped for a fair hearing, offered his co-operation, gave oral testimony before the commission. Doctors on that commission asked him to supply six case histories of the healing of incurables. Although access to medical records is not easy, Edwards did supply the number of cases sought.

He sought permission to see the findings of the doctors involved in time for him to review these findings before they were submitted to the Archbishops' Commission. He had done more than was asked for. For four weeks he tried to have his evidence heard. After several rebuffs he was told he could see the doctors' comments IF THEY FORMED PART OF THE FINAL REPORT.

It was a typical clerical move when faced with facts refuting their claims to a privileged position. Edwards realised the inquiry was now stacked against him by clerics and doctors. One of the six cases involved has already been described.

The second was of a man with cancer of the bladder—

confirmed by pathological examination. Surgery was decided upon. Edwards began the healing requested of him. Two specialists carried out the surgery. No cancer was found.

The third was a case of spinal collapse, with paralytic symptoms of the lower body. A plaster cast was applied following hospital treatment. The condition worsened. Doctors said they could do no more for him and that he could remove the plaster cast—on his own responsibility. He then called on Edwards—IN THREE MINUTES he was cured. His doctor's verdict: "A miracle". That made no difference to the doctors on the Archbishops' Commission. They had deafened their minds.

Number four was of a woman who, IN FOUR MINUTES, was cured by Edwards of a spinal deformity lasting 40 years.

Number 5 was a boy with an undiagnosed disease. From age three to ten he ate little, his body shook, he was bent double. He had been examined by many specialists and had been in five hospitals. This emaciated boy began to recover immediately Edwards initiated the absent treatment.

Number 6 was a girl with a fungoid nail growth. A doctor attending her was asked if she could be cured by spirit healing. "You will not get a miracle cure," he replied, "it is incurable." Next day she saw Edwards. Slowly the nails healed. Her doctor's comment: "I do not believe that anyone who saw these fingers ten months ago could possibly have expected them to return to normal shape."

Number 7: Parents of a girl with a growth on her neck were told by her doctors there was no known cure and that she would die. She had surgery twice and ray therapy then was sent home to die. Spirit healing cleared away the neck growth. She became vigorous. Two years later, in a hospital checkup she was found to be well.

The experts who saw her differed over the nature of the growth; all thought it was incurable.

In five of the cases cured by Edwards years had gone by. Edwards then demanded that the Archbishops' Commission make public the findings of its own medical committee in the seven cases submitted.

Said Edwards: "I regard these cases as test cases upon which my claims for spiritual healing will either stand or fall."

The archbishops are still silent, which is not unusual when they do not have a case—or a cause. Which is staggering since Anglican archbishops—and bishops, are not appointed, as far as is known, by God, but by the incumbent Prime Minister who is, in his turn, elected by the people.

It is easy to become indignant over such conduct as has been disclosed. But the subject, deepest of all human concerns, is too great, too serious, to be relegated to episcopal silence when only an honest, fair and Christian act of charity would establish a clear record.

What else must we do? The spirit world, where we are all heading, has for ages striven to aid mankind despite its follies, cruelties and hatreds because it must since the evolutionary drive impels all towards enlightenment. The answer is we do what we can, with the means available, in the circumstances prevailing. The rest will follow.

What else did Edwards' mission endure? Authority and orthodoxy are always afraid of change and challenge. Their opportunity to attack him and his work came in what, I suppose, is regarded as a public service feature on B.B.C. Television. Edwards, alone, calm, dignified, faced three antagonists who could not meet equal opposition in any cause they represented. Edwards was interrupted by the too eager inquisitors, a Scottish psychiatrist, an aggressive former politician whom I once knew when we worked on the same London newspaper, and a doctor. From personal experience I would not credit the journalist with maturity, tolerance or knowledge on healing, but with a natural verbosity which deafened reason. The medical men hid behind the decree of anonymity provided by British Medical Association decree. They were named later and are now forgotten.

You might ask: What is the worth of an opinion based on ignorance? The answer is: A B.B.C. feature on spirit healing where only one man knows and three others who don't know dominate the discussion.

The three antagonists were not at ease. Edwards answered, when he was permitted, as he always answers, the same questions with the same truths, for as Mark Twain so wisely said: An honest man does not need a good memory.

Patiently, Edwards told the Healing Story as he tells it here, as it will always be told: That doctors and scientists and chemists and other healers in the spirit world combine in a mission to help heal the human race; that when the medically-diagnosed incurables are cured the medical men, but not all of them, explain away their failures with undemonstrable excuses such as wrong diagnosis, remission, natural healing, spontaneous healing and so on with alibis bordering on the bizarre—and even foolish, as coming from men schooled in their disciplines.

Part of the discussion went this way: On statistics Edwards said that 80 percent of those seeking healing reported betterment. Cures are claimed for 20 percent of that total.

There was one incident that escaped analysis. The journalist on the programme, a brash, assertive personality, could not restrain himself. It occurred when a doctor mentioned the case of a girl cured of paralysis.

The then nameless doctor said such apparent cures were "quite common to us doctors. It is Bell's Disease, which usually clears up in six weeks."

Quietly, Edwards replied: "The doctor said he knows of cases where this happens, but our experience is that this sort of thing happens regularly with us."

The journalist, now in the spirit world, may know better if he is persuaded by his new condition. He jumped in with: "It is well known that where people are talking about themselves they are the worst possible witnesses." He was, although he did not realise it, his own "worst possible witness".

But spiritual healing does not rest upon any television programme. Only those who heal and are healed understand. In this situation, only experience counts. From our experience comes knowledge. Public forums provide matter for debate; healers produce healing and from healing we move forward to heal others until "God's will is done on earth and all is well, at last".

In a nation as homogeneous as Britain all questions are openly debated. The healing affair stirred thousands to write to Edwards protesting his treatment at the hands of two doctors and one publicist.

From a lifetime of experience of journalism I know that newspapers are the guardians of the accepted and the traditional. Hence the confusion of reporting in the Edwards situation. Newspapers blow hot and cold on such subjects as healing and evidence of Survival because of their orthodoxy and more usually because reporters assigned to cover such subjects generally know nothing of it. I had my experience with both the London and American journalists during the notorious Helen Duncan "witchcraft" trial. It was a sad situation: Ignorance sitting in judgment of knowledge.

But, taken all in all, such controversies stimulate interest whether we feel hurt because a leading figure has undergone unfair treatment. When were we ever given fair treatment? Our appeal is not to the press, radio or television. Our appeal is to reason, the only lasting criterion. Those who are healed by the spirit's agents know; the rest must choose which opinion they will follow at the moment.

Time is on our side. Each person healed is a testimonial. This will continue until opinion is on the side of the healing forces. In that day, as we change our focus from the physical to the spiritual, our societies will so change that the impetus towards knowing that there is a mental basis for physical disease will change not only medical thought but also medical practice.

That is the goal. The healers lead us towards it.

Before leaving the area of medical obstruction and controversy which is fully documented elsewhere, I offer one final case as classic for reasons that now appear:

It is a case of kyphosis (hunchback) in Elizabeth Wilson. From 1909 to 1951, or 42 years, she was treated medically and in hospital. Her spine was arched, her legs partly paralysed. She walked with two sticks and endured constant pain. She was given a spinal brace. X-ray film showed "Gross kyphosis deformity with destruction and wedging of the dorsal vertebrae". She said she would have welcomed death.

In 1951 she visited Edwards at Shere. After five minutes of treatment she said: "I felt no pain as my back moved under his hands, and the severe pain left immediately. I was able to stand upright and walk without difficulty. My balance was regained and I was able to put away my sticks. I discarded my brace."

Elizabeth Wilson, later Mrs. Oliver, walking upright, free of pain, no longer a hunchback, developed as a healer and opened a centre in Edinburgh. What did the British Medical Association say? Her cure was rejected on the ground that her condition "improved while receiving physiotherapy in addition to Mr. Edwards' ministrations."

Orthodoxy is not easily defeated, nor are Edwards and his associates. The Archbiships' Commission with its evasiveness and obfuscation, its alliance with the British Medical Association in a like effort, produced repercussions that reached culmination in two meetings, one at the Royal Albert Hall where several patients whose cures were rejected by the British Medical Association appeared as witnesses to the effectiveness of healings. Edwards declared to the cheering audience his views of the medical and clerical opposition:

"I accuse this medical committee of shameful negligence in its pretence of investigation. They did not call one patient before them. Nor did they request medical histories relating to the cases.

"Spiritual healing has not had fair play. We present the evidence for the judgment of public opinion."

He called the orthodox opposition the "unholy alliance between medicine and the Church to prevent these truths being known".

One witness only: William Olsen, a well known medium, who had been in a plaster cast because of a spinal collapse. When Olsen was being examined a specialist said to him in mockery: "What can your spirit friends do for you now?"

In one brief treatment Olsen was healed by Edwards.

That case was submitted to the Archbishops' medical committee. Their report stated: "As Mr. Olsen was healed eighteen months ago no comment can be made."

Edwards told the huge audience that reply was, "a typical excuse, evasive and fantastic".

A feature of that Royal Albert Hall meeting was the statement of the Rev. Maurice Elliott who sacrificed preferment in the church because of his active Spiritualism. He was a member of the Archbishops' Commission on Divine Healing. It also had human weaknesses for, as Elliott said:

"Harry Edwards was their main target, because of his popularity and of the great success of his unorthodox healing ministry. He had sent them a list of cases which God had healed through him. We were told that these cases had been thoroughly investigated and examined by experts on the commission and that a report had been made. We never saw that report.

"In the name of fair play, honesty and justice, I urge the Commission to send Edwards a copy of the findings of these experts. They refused to do so. The Commission sat in judgment on Christian Science and Spiritualism, which they misrepresented, distorted and ridiculed, and then condemned. How could I, who like yourselves, am a believer in fair play, honesty and justice, sign such a report? I could not and I would not."

I noticed, during the Helen Duncan "witchcraft" trial, an inscription on the central dome at the Central Criminal Court (the Old Bailey), a Latin inscription saying: "Let justice be done though the heavens fall". The heavens are still in place. The Anglican Church and its ally, the British Medical Association, are still in place—but the healing increases and will so continue until its purpose is achieved.

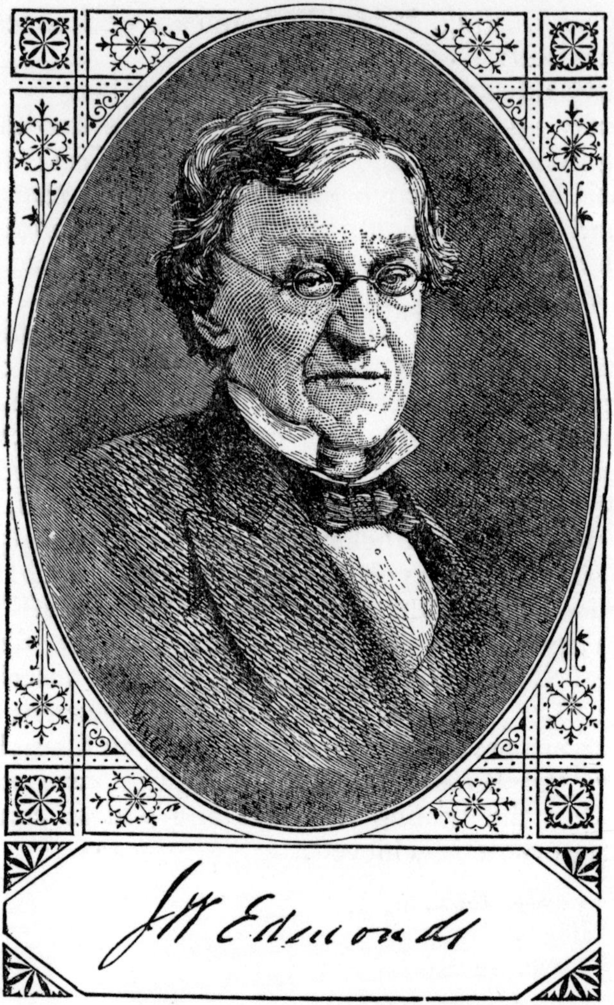

JOHN WORTH EDMONDS

Chief Justice of the Supreme Court, State of New York, was driven from the bench in 1853 because of his inquiries into Spiritualism. He had given an unpopular opinion; communication with the dead was his offence. He investigated the "Rochester Knockings" which signalled the revival of Spiritualism. A remarkable medium, he led a group of outstanding citizens in their inquiries into Survival. His articles on mediumship appeared in leading newspapers of the time.

# AMERICAN HEALERS

## High Court Judge Becomes a Medium

## Reports on Early American Healing

## The Mysterious Francis Schlatter He Healed Up to 2,000 a Day— Then Vanished

## EDMONDS

An American recorder of spirit healing in the United States was John Worth Edmonds, Chief Justice of the New York State Supreme Court, who might have become president of the United States. That was the opinion of his contemporaries. He was driven from the bench because of an outcry against an unpopular decision rendered by him. The protest was based on charges by opponents that he talked with spirits who influenced his judgments. Yet, he was respected as a jurist. No fault was found with him until he stood by his decisions.

Leading British Spiritualists of that time honoured him at a meeting in Southampton Row, London, not far from the current and a previous location of *Psychic News*. Relations between Spiritualists in both countries then were closer than they are now.

Edmonds, as becomes a learned man, kept good records before and after he was on the bench. His leaving office led to the development of his own outstanding mediumship and that of his daughter who spoke in languages she had not studied. Imagine, if a Spiritualist had become, like Lincoln, President of the United States? Edmonds was known to the leading minds of his day. At one point, he was law clerk to Martin Van Buren who later became U.S. President and who appeared to Edmonds shortly after his death.

Judge Edmonds is quoted as the source for claims that in the new world of that day, the 1850's, spirit healing was well developed. Edmonds is the chosen source of knowledge because the final 20 years of his life were devoted to Spiritualism as medium, lecturer and writer. In that day he wrote a series of articles for a leading New York newspaper that would not be published today.

Edmonds wrote, on the healing in his time:

". . . I can give nothing like an adequate idea of the vast amount of good to mankind that has flowed and is flowing from that source. For 30 years I was an invalid, varying the scene only by occasional attacks of long and severe illness. My last severe illness was in 1854 when I was sick for about four months. Then it was that the spirits came to my aid. They discovered that my disease was what no physician had suspected; but through the mediums then around me, they could not prescribe the remedy. I sent over 200 miles for one through whom they could, and whom they named to me. I followed their prescriptions from that day, and I am now in possession of better health than I have had for 40 years, or than I ever expected to enjoy."

Edmonds then summarises some successes by mediums in New York State alone by laying on hands:

> A violent pain in the side, general debility, accompanied by a most trying and nearly constant headache.
>
> In a few sittings, neuralgia of four and five months' duration, bronchitis and kidney trouble.
>
> In a few minutes a woman cured of dyspepsia and chronic diarrhoea and inflammation of the womb and bowels. A doctor said her situation was incurable.
>
> Rheumatism ended immediately by laying on hands on an adult; a child likewise healed of rheumatic fever.
>
> Various healers, all in New York State, cured: A case of "shaking palsy" which had lasted seven weeks; another healed of tuberculosis and paralysis of eight years' standing.
>
> Cures of the following diseases by laying on hands are

also listed: Spinal problems, heart disease, pressure on the brain, acute lung difficulty, cancer, blindness in one eye and partial blindness of the other, external tumour that had been growing for two years.

One healer treated from 40 to 100 patients daily, his successes including: total blindness, a club foot from birth, smallpox, scarlet and yellow fever, broken bones, insanity, children mute from birth, epileptic fits, cancers "sometimes by absorption, sometimes by removal from the body".

Judge Edmonds lived in times when orthodox religion was more powerful than it is today. As a scholar he reviewed the statements of famous men who lauded the miracles of Christianity and asked: "Now, when we reflect that healing the sick is one of the miracles referred to by these champions of Christianity, may we not ask what there is to change the character of the evidence when applied to Spiritualism?"

Several times I have referred to the 130 years history of the spirit guided effort to enlighten us as to our spiritual natures by beginning with the indispensable phenomena. But the record is longer than that. Judge Edmonds speaks from the new world in unmistakable terms. In that respect, as in others, the case is made for continuity and success in healing, mainly by those who travelled the Spiritualist way.

## SCHLATTER

One evening in July, 1895, when Alderman E. L. Fox, one of the city fathers of Denver, Colorado, U.S.A., pulled up to the fireside and opened his local paper. He caught the headlines describing the "miracles" of healing purported to have been achieved by a remarkable French-American named Francis Schlatter.

When he had read the article his mind was made up. He determined to seek Schlatter in the hope of receiving benefit for advancing deafness and the continuous pain in his side, caused by an obscure kidney disease.

The next day Fox travelled to Albuquerque, New Mexico, and traced the healer to a small adobe house in the old part of town. He found Schlatter so surrounded by visitors that the room was crowded almost to suffocation. Fox tells his own story:

"I felt from the moment I saw the healer I would be cured, and my hopes have been realised. I remained a week in Albuquerque and was convinced that not half had been told as to the powers of Schlatter. I invited him to come to Denver. I sent him a railroad ticket and he arrived in the city on the night of the August 23."

Schlatter began healing publicly in the city until September 16. From that day until November 13, when he so unexpectedly disappeared, he treated from 700 to 2,000 persons a day. Fox writes:

"Schlatter's method of treatment was unique. He took the patient by both hands which he grasped firmly and for a duration which varied according to the severity of the ailment. Most patients seemed to experience sensations which they described as resembling a slight form of electric shock.

"The sensation, when once the healer had grasped the patient's hands, commenced with a slight tremor or quiver. Then one hand would feel warm and the other cold. Prickling sensations occurred intermittently in both hands, and with them old aches and pains seemed to melt and vanish.

"As the days went by and accounts of his remarkable cures spread the crowds grew larger, and people came from all parts of the country. Eventually, local well-wishers helped him by erecting a kind of narrow gang-way, which served both to protect him from the pressure of the crowds and to enable him to treat one person at a time without difficulty.

"Standing at one end of the gangway, he received each one passing through, seizing the individual's hands in his own crossed hands, for often brief, sometimes long periods. His eyes would generally close and sometimes his lips would move as he muttered a brief, almost inaudible prayer.

"Hatless and generally without a coat, he stood there some six hours every day, treating the afflicted. Many came day after day, standing with the crowds in the street, before they were able to reach his flimsy gangway.

"Before dismissing the multitudes at the end of each day's healing, he went down among the carriages to treat the afflicted who had been brought to him, and were unable to approach by the gangway. His manner remained always serene and sympathetic, and he effected no oddity whatever beyond allowing his abundant hair to fall loosely upon his shoulders.

"Almost without variation his answer would be the same to those who thanked him: 'Don't thank me; thank the heavenly Father. Put your faith in Him, not me. I have no power but what He gives me.'

"He healed, prayed silently—and went.

"There was one other aspect of his healing which, whilst not unique, is unusual. This was a form of healing by proxy, or absent healing, by the use of handkerchiefs. In fact, some of the most remarkable of the cures effected were those achieved by these means.

"It seemed that he had only to hold a handkerchief for a few seconds when it became charged with power, as though literally healing virtue had passed through the man into the piece of material. Often Schlatter would request all patients who came to him for treatment to leave a handkerchief. This was to be used afterwards for home treatment and to ensure that healing would be continued.

"The newspapers of those times all carried full reports of the healer's remarkable work. Schlatter's cures ranged through practically all the diseases known to man. Congenital diseases, long-standing infirmity, deafness, blindness, cancer and tuberculosis. Throughout it all the healer remained unaffected by public adulation and semi-hysterical worship.

"On the night of November 13, 1895, Schlatter went to bed as usual. The evening had been full of work. Visitors from a distance had followed him home. A little before bed-time, when the visitors had gone, the family gathered around Schlatter who, as his habit was, sat down and read passages from the Bible. Then he bade me and my family goodnight and went to bed.

"It had been a fatiguing day. Thousands had passed in single file before him; and to every one in the long procession he had given the healing grasp. The skin on his fingers was worn thin. Next day the crowd was expected to be still larger.

"The following morning at six, his usual time for rising, no sound was to be heard in his room. The Fox family waited till seven then went to call him. There was no answer. I opened the door. The bed was empty. On the pillow was pinned a blank envelope. It contained a slip of paper, on which was written: 'Mr. Fox. My mission is finished and Father takes me away. Good-bye. Francis Schlatter. Nov. 13.'

"I was thunderstruck. Thousands were coming that day and the day after. But the healer had gone. No trace of him could be discovered. No one had seen him depart. The most diligent enquiries failed to reveal where he had gone.

"All that day people came, forming a great crowd outside my house. I was, at first, mute with amazement and consternation. When it swelled to thousands the silence was broken by sobs and cries, and in many cases by bitter reproaches and gibes.

"Hundreds had waited since dawn, hundreds of others arrived on the morning trains. Until late in the afternoon a pilgrimage of half-disappointed, half-hopeful people made a continuous line of returning pilgrims. Most believed that there had been some terrible mistake, that they would yet surely see the wonderful man and be healed. But as evening came on they began to turn away, hope gone, saddened by grief and disappointment."

The next day, when it became obvious that Schlatter had really vanished and there were no signs of his returning, strange scenes were witnessed outside the Fox residence. The board on which the healer stood while performing his work, part of the gangway through which patients had passed to be healed, even the fence upon which he had leaned, came to be regarded as almost sacred relics.

Men, women and children pressed forward to touch the wood with their hands or feet. Others brought handkerchiefs and pressed them to the boards. Later the alderman was warned that people were carrying away pieces of his fence, and he was forced to dismantle it and carry it into the house.

This scene did not take place in Galilee, nor did it occur in Europe in strongly Catholic countries. It happened in Denver, one of the newest cities in the United States, in the midst of the rankest materialist civilisation that any world, old or new, has ever seen.

Schlatter had always strenuously refused money in return for his healing work. It was impossible to make him accept money, and he lived only for the day with a simple and childlike faith that his wants would be met. They always were!

It was soon found that it was easy and profitable to

make money out of the healer. It is probable that it was the astuteness of the speculators, who sold places in the long line of patients to the highest bidder, that ultimately led to his departure. Places near the head of the line were sold at about two pounds each, and the bickering of the vendors sometimes grew so loud as to reach the ears of the healer.

Another characteristically smart trick was the establishment of a business in the sale of blessed handkerchiefs, which Schlatter had neither seen nor touched.

Born April 29, 1856, and reared as a Catholic at Ebershein, Alsace, France, of poor parents, Schlatter had one brother and two sisters. He left school at 14, and learned to be a shoemaker. He never married. He went to America in 1884, where he spent several years in New York working at his trade.

His unorthodox healing activities resulted, during his early years, in intermittent periods of imprisonment.

"I couldn't read the Bible in prison," he said. "They wouldn't let me have a Bible there."

At Hot Springs, Arkansas, the healer spent five and a half months in prison. In the summer of 1894 he was healing in the rugged countryside at Trockmorton, Texas, when he was taken before the local judge as a tramp. He was given the choice of leaving the town or being shut up three days in prison. Schlatter decided on this occasion that he could not cure anyone in there so he left town.

The healer's psychic powers were employed almost exclusively with healing. There was one exception, which was recorded at the time in several Denver newspapers.

As the long procession of patients filed past the healer, he startled everyone by saying, quietly but firmly, to a man who asked for treatment, "You are a murderer." The voice of the healer was not raised but the words seemed to penetrate a great area of the crowd about him.

The healer commanded the man to pass. He refused, and insisted that he should be treated.

"I cannot treat you," said the healer in low, firm tones.

"Why?" insisted the man.

"Shall I tell you—do you desire me to tell you right here, before all these people?" asked the healer.

"Yes," said the man impudently.

"I cannot treat you; you are a murderer!"

Whether the man accused was a resident of that town or a stranger is not known. Where he came from was as deep a mystery as where he went. Within five minutes dozens of men were looking for him. But the man who slipped away in the crowds around the healer was never traced.

There must have been many healers whose missions, if not as colourful as Schlatter's, were as effective. Apart from the mystery of his coming and going, there remains the method of applying healing—the laying on of his hands, the conditioning of handkerchiefs and the absent healing. Schlatter would occupy a high place in any healers' hall of fame, as would many others who are now as obscure as he was.

# WHY SOME HEALINGS FAIL

Since much is written of the revolutionary views emerging from direct experience of healing from spiritual sources, sceptics and inquiring souls logically ask: since so much healing succeeds, why are there failures?

There is no point to be made here for the statistical, classic, clinical answer that truth, or a semblance of it, is a matter of percentages. On such a foundation the claims and facts of spiritual healing do not rest, although these factors may be used in assessing the evidence for the spirit healing.

The answer comes from the science and art of spirit healing itself and is now expressed in these words from a spirit source in answer to the question: "Why does spirit healing sometimes fail?"

There is no need to qualify the word fail as though it were a rebuke or an admission of wrongdoing or sin, or inadequacy. In all of mankind's endeavours there are failures—and successes.

In seeking to discover something of the art of living in a complex body within a complex society, it would be beyond reason and the reign of natural law if we passed an entire lifespan without failure, that is, non-accomplishment of our wishes and desires, our dreams and ambitions.

For what most often we call failure is as important as what we call success, that lure and trap for the spiritually unwary among us, who are self-deceived into believing that whatever they desire is best for them at all times and that what causes discomfort, yes, and even the distressing pain of disease, is the mark and sign of failure.

In such case we but speak of frustration, an element of the law of spiritual growth.

If there were no failures there could not be successes since the two states are but the sides of the coin and currency of our efforts to evolve. Only those who most know pain in themselves can best understand it in others since the experience of pain is registered in the soul, the only imperishable aspect of ourselves.

Since pain comes to all at some time, and with others is a burden borne throughout a whole lifetime, we are in the presence of an absolute, or as close to it as we may come while we express ourselves through the flesh.

Pain speaks to us of natural and spiritual laws broken somewhere, at some time. Nature's memory of breaches of her laws is perfect; our recollections of the state and nature of the causes of pain and suffering are imperfect, hence mankind cries its pain to the silence wherein broods the secret of amending our sorrows and from the darkness brings such light as healers may give in their lives of service.

Now comes the heart-aching question: Then is healing a breach of law since often it succeds in ending pain? Should we not suffer for ever? Are healers imitating what many say are God's laws when the lame, the halt, the blind and others so distressed that they pray for death's soothing embrace and for nature's sweet, sweet sleep—and cannot be healed?

The answer must be, or the heavens shall fall, that healing follows upon obedience to the spiritual laws by which we breathe, move, love and suffer. When the spiritual clock of our lives strikes the appointed hour in our evolution, healer and sufferer are brought together. This is a study beyond our capacity.

Relief of pain may come by the healing touch, by the

soothing word, by the distant flight of healing power transmitted from its spiritual reservoirs to those who have called out, mostly in the silence, for relief.

When the soul in pain is ready to receive, when the healer is attuned, when the healing spirits in the real world of the invisible have developed the knowledge, when time is conjoined with circumstance, the subtle, silent, invisible spirit power strikes at the disease—then pain must cease.

All healing is revelation of the power of the spirit. That is its mission beyond pain's ceasing.

Again, the question comes: Then why are there failures? Because the entire circumstances are not present for success. The thoughtful inquirer will, if the foregoing is true, develop his own thoughts, but the kernel is in the nut. A prophet and seer has said: Whether there be prophecies they shall also fail; itself a prophecy. He might also have said: where there are healings some shall fail; itself a prophecy.

If all who suffer and cry for relief were to be healed before the next coming dawn, we, the human race, would in measurable time and known circumstances once again develop the conditions which give birth to what we know as disease. And that is not prophecy but certainty since we still live and grow in the world of the fallible, the largely undeveloped. When we are ready, when we have grown to greater awareness of our spiritual potential, we will live by the laws of life and will cease our transgressions which make our way hard.

Healing is a mission of relief for we who break the laws of life. Healing is teaching of the laws of life. When we know what truly we are, the healing of the nations will be a success since we will not transgress since we will know that is the path of our failure to live by the spirit.

By wisdom for ourselves and compassion for others we

will change our world to the point where healing itself will be restored to its proper place as an integral gift of our natures and not the emergency service it is now. Then and only then will we say there are no healing failures, since in that far distant time we will, largely, have evolved beyond disease of soul, mind and body.

Disease is not a punishment for wrongdoing, nor a curse for lack of belief or breach of any of the many taboos society has developed on its crab-like course in evolution. Disease is not a penalty under the man-made crime called sin; disease is a consequence of certain specified acts which arise from like thoughts and emotions. The cause unleashed, the consequences follow, else there is no reason in nature, the garment worn by spirit that we may recognise that Wondrous One.

There is no means yet discovered by which we can escape ourselves or the results of our impact on everything we meet. In other times, less educated, crude but close to the earth's dominion, men—and women—devised charms to modify and then, presumably, to counteract the effects of what we do. We, of this sophisticated age, have devised our own "charms", a range of poisons, physical, mental and emotional, in our search for release from the hells we create.

In due time, now or later, in body, soul and spirit, we must act to correct the adverse conditions we establish by our slow, suicidal acts. If you argue that you do not accept that view, nature has no counter-position. Time and the facts will tell. But, when once we recognise that we must begin to rectify the wrongs we do to others—and ourselves—then the silent, subtle healing begins until, one day, we say we are cured. The spirit has triumphed; man, the prodigal son, returns to his Father's house and he may now go on his spiritual way, rejoicing.

# A SPIRIT'S VIEW OF HEALING

That view of the relationships between the successes and failures in spiritual healing is derived from a spirit source, as is the following expression from that widely beloved teacher in the spirit, Silver Birch. He is, as we who know him well, a teacher of penetrating power derived, as he says, from much experience and from those whom he, in turn, serves. As with others of his brotherhood, he masks his identity behind the name of a tree, much as an American Indian might. That is a discussion for other times.

We are presently enmeshed in the net of circumstance in which knowledge of healing comes slowly into the thinking of mankind.

So, my wife and I, responding to that invisible teacher, Silver Birch, talked with him to learn his views of healing, since much of his contact with us earth dwellers is in counselling mediums of all kinds. He is, in truth, a healer of souls. His eloquence is unequalled, his patience has no end, his gentle firmness is felt where the exchanges stray from their courses.

Since we had already received the foregoing spirit view of the nature of failure in some healing, Silver Birch was asked to comment on the nature of healing.

For those who have never attended what is called a seance, or meeting for spirit communion, maybe a brief description will set the scene. In a small flat in London the medium, Maurice Barbanell, and his wife, Sylvia, my wife, Fay, and I sit in good light. The medium relaxes, we are quiet. As he has done thousands of times before, the medium appears to fall asleep. Presently through his lips we hear a voice far different from his, a greeting from the invisible. The medium's voice is light; the voice of the invisible spirit teacher deeper and of an unidentified kind. He once told us it was a voice established for his work. There followed a prayer to the Great Spirit, the invariable opening, and at once the Indian, as he says he is and is named for a tree, greets us, and speaks an eloquent and moving prayer.

Much of the session is in the nature of students with some post-graduate experience refreshing their wisdom with their teacher. I put the questions on the meaning and purpose of healing. This is his answer, given without notice, without a moment's hesitation:

The purpose of spiritual healing is to enable divine power to produce, firstly, a physical or mental result, and also a spiritual result. Without the spiritual result, however successful the physical or mental healing may be, it has failed in its purpose.

Healing, like all the phenomena of what is called mediumship, is intended to draw attention to the fundamentals of life which are the spiritual realities.

In brief, the object of healing is to touch the sufferer's soul so that it can begin to come into its own. Sickness should be the means of making that individual aware of what lies beyond the physical senses. That is the prime objective of the healing.

I don't have to tell you that healing, the power of healing, emanates from the Supreme Power, the Great Spirit.

So, briefly, it can be said the power comes from spirit through the spirit that is the gift of the spirit to heal the spirit which is that of the patient. All the way through it is completely a spiritual exercise.

Now, the great contribution that Edwards has made is

to reduce the healing to its essence of simplicity so that there is no need for ritual or ceremony, for magnetic passes to be made, hands to be washed before and after every treatment or long phases of meditation to be pursued before the healing, but to achieve such a degree of attunement that the power flows in the greatest possible force through the instrument. It is divine in its origin.

The future healing must consist in the development of that attunement. Progressively, attainment will mean greater attunement and greater attunement will mean greater attainment.

Edwards is, in essence, a pioneer who becomes a lesson and an example for others to follow to show what can be achieved when there is a completely dedicated human instrument and a close attunement with the power of the spirit. It will spread in many lands and bring awareness to many people that the power of the spirit is a reality, that they are primarily spiritual beings with bodies, not bodies with spirits, that there is an overall, divine, supreme power that regulates and controls all life, all destiny, all that is, all that has been, all that ever will be.

That is as I see it.

# THE PROSPECT BEFORE US

K*

Together we began this healing story with an inquiry into the cause of crises in man's journey from his spirit home to his experience in this world as preparation for return, tried and seasoned by all that nature and his destiny can impose upon him. In the world's philosophies there are no such claims. Our premise is simple: We all are souls since that is what we are created; expressions of an unending power named in many tongues, experienced in everything and designed for continuing fulfilment.

There are creeds which announce a specific time of creation. There are others which ignore inquiry into beginnings and take their stands upon an assumption that there are two states of being; life and non-life. Into such matters we do not venture since the ages have not yet produced any evidence that there was a beginning. The non-life people find their views satisfying because they are thereby relieved of the need to answer the questions asked before: what are we; where or from which condition do we come; why is life on earth so difficult; where and into which condition do we go when our days of trial and error are ended with a cry, a sigh or a blessed sleep and forgetting?

We, who supposedly emerge from nothing but matter, develop in such complexity that we are amazed at the wonders within yet can explain nothing of the why and how of life but deal only with the living present and hope for light when we have done with the body.

Most of our days are lived in the world of matter. That is the basis of science which finds itself now confronted with other serious considerations.

The continuing references to science are unavoidable since it is the single most powerful shaper of thought in our days. How often do we state "Science says"? Science says many things but is always changing its views as discoveries change opinion. Science has achieved its eminence by mind—power since formal religion cannot explain as much or as satisfactorily as science does. Public opinion flows where thought has made a channel. There is nothing new in formal religion since it long ago declared its possession and dispensing of the truth and made its voice heard on all matters of public interest and consequence.

Much of the world goes about its business of evolution without the slightest regard for the mere opinions of churches, which is not the same as saying that individuals within the churches are not progressive.

All of mankind is daily involved in the consequences of science applied, not necessarily in scientific theories.

We are concerned to present a picture to show how all that has gone before is part of an evolution. Since formal religion lacks inspiration and revelation, mankind has shifted its loyalty to technology: the art of doing something with the discoveries of science. Indeed, technology now dominates our lives: the genie of science is out of the bottle and provides us, among other benefits, with the means of rapid, total destruction or death by slower, more precise, more widespread pollution at all levels.

It is necessary now to call only one witness to testify as to the power and future of science. Witnesses for the spirit view of life have already testified. Both views are supported by facts. The spirit view does not contradict the scientific but it prevails since it reveals facts not yet faced by science. And the spirit does cross the boundary between the physical and the metaphysical, while science, so far, is isolated by its own choice.

Our witness now is Max Planck, a revered figure in the science community, second only to Einstein for his discoveries. In his long life—he died nearly 90 years old —he changed thought in his field. His story is similar to that of non-conforming Sir Alfred Russel Wallace. The great men of science in his day ignored Planck. He had what his eulogist said was an "inner call". He solved problems which defeated many others. We non-scientific people do not grasp the impact of his achievements—the principal one being his theory of the law of radiation, or the quantum theory. He suffered much from academic opposition before achieving his contribution to science which of itself has little relevance to this summation; it is mentioned to confirm Planck's eminence and for his views on the Other World. (The quantum theory is that energy is not absorbed and radiated continuously but discontinuously in definite units or quanta, like a pulsation instead of an unbroken stream.)

Planck speaks of the role of science as "exploration of the outside world"—or the way we receive impressions from the senses. Information so received differs from person to person and is modified or elaborated as our experience increases.

Then he arrives at natural laws—the same for all races and nations and, I add, in all times—a true absolute in the scientific sense. If so, why and how, then, the diversities, divisions and problems? We have no argument about the necessity for air, food, water, shelter and so on.

Planck talks of the "real world", the sense world which gave science a solid base until it was seen that even atoms change. In a universe of change why would even atoms be exempt?

In short, Planck shows us the evolution of scientific

theory from the sensory, the absolute, to new absolutes—the theory of Relativity and of his major discoveries in radiation. He foresaw the time when the discoveries of this era will be regarded as not so absolute in light of increasing knowledge.

He talks of phenomena based upon experience through the senses yet he says:

"As there is a material object behind every sensation, so there is a metaphysical reality behind every thing that human experience shows to be real." He explains that "behind" might as well be stated as "in" or "within", adding: "Nature is neither core nor shell—she is everything at once. The essential point is that the world of sensation is not the only world which may conceivably exist, but that there is still another world. To be sure, this other world is not directly accessible to us, but its existence is indicated time and again, with compelling clarity, not only in practical life, but by the labours of science."

It is noteworthy that the more eminent the scientist the more mystical he becomes.

> Planck speaks of the ". . . gaping chasm . . . between the real world of phenomena and the real world of metaphysics . . . But at the same time we catch here a glimpse of the boundaries which exact science is unable to cross."

Exact science depends upon the physical wholly and must, to be admitted as being established, conform to measurements for exactness. Elsewhere Planck says that only as older scientists die, do the younger men and women come to receive views their predecessors rejected.

That sounds familiar.

Space is given Planck because of his eminence and frankness in approaching the metaphysical question.

We have seen already that scientists are almost religious in their orthodoxy, yet some of them accept the phenomena of the psychic world but pay little or no attention to the human world. Even Planck says we learn through the body alone. If so, where did his theories come from? He does not deal with that position and nowhere suggests any awareness of the psychic world while stating the mystic's affirmation of the "within".

In the healing story it is shown that there is no problem of unreal versus real worlds. To repeat a basic concept, as taught from the spirit realm—all worlds are one. Because our communication is, in a sense, not a continuous stream but is pulse-like, we have our own, psychic quantum theory of crossing the chasm to which Planck refers.

In our own real world we cross the chasm across which there is an invisible bridge, else we could not dream, experience visions, enjoy communication with our spirit friends and teachers, receive inspiration and, as is amply proved, healing.

It is because most scientists and others refuse to investigate that much is withheld from those who want to know but cannot find the knowledge.

It is a question for the future whether scientists generally will reach that point in discovery where they achieve at the physical level what is already achieved by healers who are wholly dependent upon spirit power and spirit beings for their achievements. So far, in all the decades that have elapsed since healing came into prominence, there has not been developed a physical equivalent. If, for example, doctors could demonstrate a group of healings of the kind offered by Edwards and others, without spirit direction, then they would be in a superior position; then indeed the medical arts would be revolutionised. But they are not even on the road to that position although some of the more venturesome are finding it difficult to ignore the imperative need to admit the case for the reality of a spiritual world.

Spirit healers do not conduct experiments in, say, radiation, as did Planck, yet they demonstrate cures that, theoretically, are achieved by some form of radiation.

The healers cannot "turn on" the healing force at will, despite any claims to do so. Yet they show proof of being channels, vehicles, instruments or any other term that may be used to state the distinction between the effects of healing and its cause, or causes.

Thus, we have the two worlds, the two sciences and arts; the physical and the metaphysical. When we have made a sufficient impact on public opinion with our services and in our teaching to inform any who care to listen to the truths of the spirit, there will be changes in public and scientific opinion upon healing and other basic matters.

Healing is not the end; it is the beginning of new views of life, consciousness and society. Healing is also teaching of the spirit; teaching is also a prime mode of healing: the two are one.

Elsewhere the question has been discussed: Why is there so much disease? Since we no longer deal in demonology, disease cannot be ascribed to malevolent or sinister influences to be exorcised by the crudities or brutalities of the ages of superstition. We have to deal rationally with disease not only in the terms employed by physical medicine and the related services, public and private, but as seen from the spirit world whence the healing originates.

With the growing exception of those doctors who ascribe much disease to a mental and emotional source, the movement of modern medicine is toward repair, refinement in procedures, greater instrumentation, "spare parts", increase in drug research—and more hospitals; all to cope with more disease and more deaths from disease. Costs rise disproportionately to the increase in the total of diseased persons.

There appears to be no term to cancer research. From some of the reports that escape from time to time from the vast array of establishments where cancer is studied and treated, it appears to have long since taken on the ways of industry. Any activity that has endured so long must, by sheer weight of money and numbers, become a heavily vested interest.

There is some light. More physicians have turned to the question of thought applied by the patients to themselves as a form of therapy. Should this departure from established therapies succeed, even to a minor degree, it is logical to anticipate an outbreak of cynicism from the orthodox interests in the world of cancer research. Those who know of the effectiveness of spirit healing in the cure of cancer must welcome the development of self-applied thought.

The time is long past when such healers as psychiatrists and others in mental healing should have been recruited to help deal with the cancer problem. We, who know what is done by spirit healing, long since recognised the value of the unstressed mind for relieving then curing all manner of diseases. Indeed, the first awareness of a turn in the road from distress to the commencement of healing is a relaxation of tension.

The connection between that proved fact and reports of psychiatry as a form of therapy in treatment of cancer are encouraging. It does not matter what group adopts the mental approach so long as it is maintained, since, once upon that road, many with the healing potential will develop and add to the healing army.

In such fashion the healing service will grow as the Democracy of Healing is established in the public mind. It could not be otherwise; the healing gift had to be widely discovered since the foundations were well laid by the pioneers and cannot now be destroyed. Healing is at least as important as space flight, atomic power stations, huge armies and all the other designs for consuming the fruits of mankind's labours.

Among other advantages and boons arising from the growth of the Democracy of Healing is that its cost is minimal since the healers, with few exceptions, serve as volunteers. Also, spirit healing does not require building of hospitals, nor expensive equipment, nor huge staffs. The reader can take the point from there.

We turn now to the social consequences of healing since it is held that the spirit mission is not intended alone for the cure of physical and mental disease. While disease cannot be the only consequence of society's misdeeds, there is ample evidence to produce an indictment of such proportions as to ensure certain conviction under any system of law; we are imbrued with society's misdeeds yet we are society.

All disease comes to a climax in the person, even in epidemics. While it is rare that we mourn long for a disaster, a death in the family, even from disease, strikes home, even to the most disciplined and self-contained.

In this western world mainly we have but to extend our minds a little to become aware of the twofold benefits provided almost without cost—evidence and proof of Survival and evidence and proof that spirit healing is here to serve mankind.

Some time will pass before the fuller effects will be recognised as established elements of a changed society, a quieter society which will have learned to live harmoniously within each soul and within the society as a whole. We are inured to regard disease as inevitable, with fear and stress as part of the natural flow of events and death as a tragedy from which there is neither escape nor meaning.

Man, who may learn to discipline himself gently to live in full health, is learning to restrain the effects of his terrifying power to reproduce. The consequences of rivers of children arriving on earth unaccompanied by oceans of food and other necessities has resulted in another signpost being passed. We learn most by suffering; seldom by forethought, but we are learning that we are on the brink of much self-inflicted disaster. We now act not out of prudence but fear—of want.

References here to the planned development for mankind call for discussion. The statements already made are clear. The perceptive person will, in wonder, ask what authority is there for such claims? The spirit communicators point to their records and to the records of those who preceded them in their roles. They point to the steady decline of loyalty to the authoritarian religions, to the changed views of death and Survival, to the reforms in many societies, to the advances in thought in all areas of human concern and welfare in the direction of lessening fear and increasing confidence.

It is claimed that concern for the deprived, the unfortunate and the less well endowed mentally and physically is due to the inspiring of souls ready to urge such reforms once considered radical and dangerous but now accepted as commonplace and ripe for extension. The trend is toward democracy in all things at all levels, embracing as far as persuasion may prevail, the basic elements of our societies. It is almost a cliche that we humans take three steps forward, two backward and one sideways—yet we improve, slowly.

The massive ignorance inspired by superstition has yielded to education; the sciences have continued to extend thought. The principal problems are not within nature but in man. Nature provides sufficient for all—when justice is done. For justice to be done we must recognise its imperative. Justice denied produces social disease which breeds disease in the individual for justice denied is frustration—the breeder of cancer and other ills.

The power of orthodox religion had to be disarmed. The power of armed forces will lessen as we are persuaded that killing bodies is not the same as killing souls. Bodies perish. Even so, souls are safe from all weapons; the only retardants of soul growth are fear, greed, injustice, hate and exploitation.

Once persuade a majority that survival of bodily death is a natural fact and man will tend to be less fearful. His cause for fear will have gone.

Once prove to a majority that spirit healing and spirit evidence of Survival are truths and we have the foundations for a new vision, a new song of life on earth.

What other changes shall we see: that there will be a new psychology since the soul and the psychic nature will be known and, to a degree, understood. In that coming day the new psychologists will, with understanding of the true nature of man, teach rather than preach the techniques of living the fuller life. We must cease the production of the spiritually, physically and bodily handicapped. We will, in time, reshape our methods of education since we will know what we are educating—the soul—so that it may achieve its fullest expression while increasing its ability to live in harmony with nature and its fellows.

You will say, silently, that this is utopian. There is nothing to make utopia undesirable nor unrealisable; utopia was only a limited glimpse into the future. And, what do we have now that could not be vastly improved without hurt to any save those who do not look beyond the material life?

The coming more spiritualised person will not tolerate the environments that pollute nature—and man. The goal is a world without fear since it will live by a philosophy that sees life as continuous and not as a contest against forces we do not understand—and fear.

This is no vision of races of the ultra-good spending

their days shouting hosannas; it is a forecast of what must come as a result of the disclosure of the forces now influencing all races, everywhere. It is natural that the most progressive nations will take the lead, not the domination, since that would more deeply entrench the wrongs that produce so much disease.

It was necessary that, in layman's language, the impact of scientific thought on society should be examined so far as it concerned our two main interests, Survival and healing. All scientists are not equally concerned about the welfare of man; the life interests of many are so absorbing that newer concepts in other fields are unwelcome intrusions. But there are outstanding women and men who shape world thought. Each advance of a major nature modifies society to the degree that either new technology develops or philosophies change. No discovery has ever disproved or even provided a challenge to the claims set out in the evidence for Survival, and later of the evidence of healing from a conscious, intelligent spirit source.

If we look back we will see that from the time in which Planck was at work upon what became, for science, a major discovery, that even he who recognised the limits of his profession, had nothing to offer as a means of entering the metaphysical dimension he foresaw from what he had achieved. He proposed a theory—in science a requirement—and neglected to suggest a means of demonstrating its validity for all mankind. This is not a matter alone for the laboratory and the study; for exchanges of views with other learned women and men but an essential knowledge for all souls. These have a right to know factually of that "other world" of which Planck writes and in which he now lives and grows. What would he say if he could again communicate as freely and as frankly as he did in his scientific autobiography? What is it in us that prevents the mind from reaching out to know what has always existed? I hesitate to state the view that some are ready to take such a step and some are not; it is a matter of choice since the opportunity exists from the moment we perceive that matter is not enough either as a view or as a basis for the kinds of societies we have endured for so many centuries and under such heavy burdens.

The years between Planck's discoveries and the current views have not been filled with news of scientific study of the import of his views on the metaphysical. Other Worlds, his theory of radiation, it appears, is enough: it is closest to the material: it may be adaptable to a technological opportunity; it may, in the long run, give rise to a new industry, beneficial, hopefully, and harming none.

Is there no place in the world of science for thought beyond the material? While science neglects its duty to look into the Other World the market place of ideas is deprived of its greatest commodity—the liberating truth of Survival.

Come now to consider the judgment of a Nobel Prize winner, Prof. Luria, who retreated from his opportunity to take one step beyond the brain considered as the mind. His skills and insights impress his peers, yet he continued on the path of "more biology, more biology". Has more biology succeeded in the cases of cancer, arthritis and other diseases? Must scientists continue in the same circular track left by pioneers?

There was a time before Galen when little was known of anatomy. Research led to knowledge, of course, and treatment followed. But which biology will yield us the final secret of the origin of thought? Biology of the brain? The thoughtful person will develop his own views from that situation. Materialism still holds sway among the orthodox; they are twins.

The only developments in coming to grips with the

brain-mind question have occurred in the psychic and spiritual field. Because that body of knowledge is not developed as a result of academic training it is suspect and disregarded.

From Planck to Luria the path of not knowing is clear. Planck was made aware by the mathematics of his dilemma; Luria is impressed by the ultra-mathematics of the brain/mind, and prefers to seek in the brain the secrets of the origins of thought—not yet of life itself.

But for the discoveries of those pioneering scientists who proved the existence of the Other World, this world would have become more materialistic since materialism has proved its power of survival. Matter is real; it is not all.

In such a circumstance the art or application of spirit-directed healing, based upon spirit science, was brought forward to aid humanity in taking the inevitable step from the material to the spiritual. I trust that position is now clear after so many words, so many factual reports and so many illustrations.

It is remarkable that in the earlier days of the renewal of awareness of the spirit, there were leading scientists who found truths through studies of phenomena—the path stated by Planck. When that task was done, the movement was and continues phenomenal. From physical phenomena, where it all begins, we moved to mental phenomena, to demonstrations yielding results that science has not even now begun to study seriously. For them Planck's radiation was enough; his Other World remains a statement understood by Spiritualists and their like because he stated what they know.

Since we cannot rely upon either orthodox science or orthodox religion to enlighten the public mind on these essential studies, we have had and will always have the human exponents drawn from the democracies of humanity. No matter how powerful we may become as individuals, we are still members of the spiritual democracy called humanity. It is from that source that the medium/healers, trance speakers, clairvoyants and clairaudients come; the counsellors and writers. It is to develop a spiritual democracy that they serve.

No searchlight is required to discover where the greatest opportunities for developing that trend exist. We have but to look around us. Present difficulties do not invalidate the future. The power is available to heal and teach. Nothing that we may do can prevent that force from its fuller expression as more and more volunteer to serve. In serving others we serve our own progress. What was mystery in the healing art and science is become regular practice. By doing, healers learn; by learning they become more proficient. Being known by their service, their effect upon opinion increases. Thus are the seeds sown of the coming Democracy of the Spirit.

The way of the pathfinders is hard; the goal glorious and the joy they bring with their healing beyond all that the attractive material offers. Healing prospers Healers: they rejoice in healing. Can more be desired?

It is certain as the sunrise, in a world of uncertainties made by man, that the opening words telling of man's anguish and pain and crises have not led us to deeper despair. To map the country we are to dwell in for a time is to ensure we will find our way. That is the purpose of this story: to show a way from ignorance of spirit with its eternal, natural laws, to states of consciousness, and to societies where these laws are the bases of life as near as we can devise, and that where we lack our fellow spirits in that other world will inspire us to supply.

There is no other aim: if a truth is told here the work is justified: if it is not so, then mankind has still before it the choice of a world in continuing crisis until a condition of chaos develops for which there is no remedy—and nature must take its course.

The foundations of the Democracy of the Spirit were laid long ago. Many attempts have been made to destroy them. Even more attempts have been made to complete the structure. Men fail; the spirit does not fail. We cry complaining when we suffer the blows we aim at one another since the law is as perfect as any law of science is said to be.

No one seer or prophet may discern the whole likeness of what is to come. Nature blesses us with memory and mercifully balances it with a forgetting. As Paul said: Now we see in part . . . then in full. But we have a foreview because we work as with hammer and anvil to shape it. We see not shadows but substance and from that substance—thought—we shape our ideas, our lives, our laws, and sow such seed from ourselves as may bring forth such children as will live free of fear, directed by knowledge, and dedicated to serve those who are less in substance but the same as being created equally, all, all of the one spirit of life which has no beginning and no end.

# FUNDAMENTAL POSTULATES THAT GOVERN SPIRITUAL HEALING

The source of spiritual healing is God, Who created the perfect laws that govern life. Sickness follows the transgression of these laws.

The purpose of spiritual healing is to stimulate man's latent divinity, so that he lives in harmony with God's laws and automatically reaping the result, fulfils the reason for earthly life.

Spiritual healing, therefore, helps to accomplish the divine intention for man's spiritual progress.

The postulates that follow are concerned with the fulfilment of the divine purpose.

Every change in the universe is the result of law-governed forces. Nothing takes place by chance or without a reason. Thus our bodies are subject to definite laws which control our health from birth to the grave.

1. *Spiritual healing is the result of law-governed healing forces that induce change.*

*Purposefully* to effect any change, intelligent direction is needed to administer the law-governed forces to the subject.

Example: Man must direct the force of electricity to produce a *given* result within the laws which govern that force.

2. *The effective administering of a healing force requires intelligent direction.*

Through spiritual healing, "incurable" patients are

cured. The term "incurable" signifies that medicine can do no more, that earthly wisdom is exhausted, and the patient is condemned to suffer without hope of recovery. Thus when a spiritual healing succeeds with an "incurable", it denotes that a wiser intelligence than that of man is responsible for the law-governed, ordered change. If this intelligence is not earthly, then it must be non-material.

3. *The intelligent direction of a healing force originates from the spirit realm.*

A diversity of human ills, from mental sickness to cancer, from nervous breakdowns to cataract, from blue babies to arthritis, are successfully treated by spiritual healing. This denotes that the directing intelligence is able to diagnose the cause of the affliction and to determine the correct character and strength of the healing force needed to remedy each given condition.

4. *In a successful healing, the directing intelligence is able to ascertain the cause of disease and knows how to administer the remedial force to induce a state of beneficial change within the patient.*

## THE LAWS

There are some physical laws which control the material world. As there must be order in spirit life there are spirit laws. The administering of a spirit. healing force must conform to its laws, just as physical laws govern physical forces.

5. *The physical and spirit laws combined come within the definition of the total law.*

6. *No healing is possible outside the confines of the total law.*

*Contact Healing:* It is a law that harmony must exist between transmission of a force and its conscious or unconscious reception. Furthermore, the receiver must be in attunement with the transmitter.

7. *The intelligently directed healing forces emanate from a non-physical realm, therefore, they are not physical, but through healership are transformed into physical effects.*

8. *In contact healing the healer is the attuned receiver through whom the spirit healing forces are received for transmission to the patient.*

9. *One function of the healer is to be the means, where necessary, for non-physical energy to be made physical.*

10. *The patient's spirit self can act as a receiver and transformer of healing force, in contact healing as well as in absent healing.*

*Absent Healing:*

*When absent healing is effective, attunement is established between the healing intelligence and the patient.*

11. *The healer's function is to be the communicative link between the absent patient and the healing source.*

Every person has a spirit nature which can be in attunement with spirit intelligence. He is, therefore, able to receive spirit direction and healing forces.

12. *In absent healing, the patient's spirit self acts as the transformer, and receiver of healing forces through his spirit nature.*

13. *The patient's spirit nature is able to receive corrective thoughts and directives from the healing intelligence rightly to influence him and so overcome primary causes of disease.*

## THE HEALING FORCES

For the alleviation and healing of physical ill-effects the healing forces produce a changed chemical effect in the patient's body. This implies a profound spirit knowledge of chemistry and energies.

14. *The spirit healing forces, producing a planned chemical change, must, before the act of transformation, be synonymous with the energy-formations comprising physical matter.*

15. *These healing forces are able to create chemical changes through the application of one given form of energy to another.*

16. *Beneficial chemical changes are also induced through the physical bodily intelligence.*

17. *The healing forces possess individual, particularised characteristics to effect beneficial change through introducing new factors that alter to disperse the harmful conditions.*

In cases of direct dispersal or induced chemical change, the effects are directed to the disharmony alone, and there is no interference with the healthy tissue or structure.

18. *This implies that the spirit intelligence performs an exact process, influencing only diseased cells or structures, without disturbing the healthy ones.*

## TWO QUESTIONS

*Question No.* 1. Why does spirit healing fail to achieve success in some cases?

*Question No.* 2. Why are there sometimes recessions after cures have taken place?

### *ANSWERS TO QUESTION No.* 1.

In considering this problem, we are in the realm of imponderables. All spirit healing is law-governed. It is part of the natural law that every individual must die. No spirit healing can confer earthly immortality. Even, however, in cases regarded as failures because of death's inevitability, it is certain that many patients have been relieved of much suffering. They also receive an inner peace which helps the process of transition.

We still know very little about the way in which spirit healing works. We do know that its source is divine, and therefore spiritual. Its power comes through the healer's spirit body and achieves success by stimulating the patient's natural recuperative processes which are part of his spiritual life force. Thus, healing can be briefly summarized as from spirit, through spirit, to spirit.

The spirit operators are constantly experimenting with the healing power they transmit. Though infinite in its source, it is transmitted at varying levels conditioned by the spiritual development of the healer and the patient. Healing is accomplished through vibrations or radiations. Thus a patient may fail with one healer and succeed with another, depending on the harmony, or lack of it, between them at the time of treatment.

The spirit "know-how" based on experience and trial and error is constantly increasing. This is shown by the fact that speedier results are obtained with some ailments than was the case many years ago. It may well be that in future there will be successes with types of ailment that are failures to-day.

The whole essence of spirit healing is to awaken and stimulate the patient's spiritual nature. Bodily conditions are usually symptoms and not causes. Where the patient's spiritual nature, for one reason or another, cannot be aroused, and the cause of the disease has a spiritual origin, there may be apparent failure. There will also be fewer failures as healers live more dedicated lives. While healing is a natural gift, its quality is dependent upon the healer's character, moral growth and spiritual development.

Healing cannot replace what has been removed by surgery, such as an amputated finger. Nor can it restore, for example, nerves that have disappeared after meningitis has taken its toll. Nevertheless, healing can often produce amelioration.

There are, unfortunately, some patients who do not want to get well. They seem to enjoy their self-imposed martyrdom and resist the healing by persistently maintaining their conditions by anticipatory thinking.

*ANSWER TO QUESTION No.* 2.

The answer to both questions is largely to be found in the fact that patients perpetuate the physical, mental and possibly spiritual causes of their ailments. The effect of healing should be that the patients change their way of life. If they resume the dietary conditions or live in dampness or continue with wrong thinking, which were responsible for their ailments, then there will be recessions.

Another reason for recession is the patient's inability to recognize, for example, that his joints are no longer locked. He has lived with this condition for so many years that he cannot mentally free himself, with the result that this causes joints to lock again.

Another cause may be when patients discharge themselves before the course has been completed.